CW00923531

Greener Pa
Brown Blazers

Edna Hunneysett

chipmunkapublishing
the mental health publisher

Edna Hunneysett

Published by
Chipmunkapublishing
United Kingdom

http://www.chipmunkapublishing.com

Copyright © 2020 Edna Hunneysett

ISBN   978-1-78382-540-0

About the Author

Edna Mary Hunneysett was born in 1940 near Stratford-upon-Avon, but in her infancy, the family moved to a small, remote farm on the North Yorkshire moors where Edna, the third of seven children, spent her early life. After passing the eleven plus exam, she was a boarder at a convent grammar school. On finishing school, she was employed by the Inland Revenue. She married in 1961 and has eight children, twenty-one grandchildren and three great grandchildren. From 1977 to 1991, she worked part-time at a BBC local radio station. She gained a BA Hons (Div) in 1995 and an MA in 1998. She lives with her husband, a retired teacher, in Middlesbrough.

Also by Edna Hunneysett

Our Suicidal Children: Where Are You, God?
Pastoral Care: Mental Health
From The Heart: Mental Health
Greener Beyond The Hill

Acknowledgements

Many thanks to our daughter, Stephanie, who, having taught English for years, helped me immensely with advice and suggestions after painstakingly reading my manuscript. I am indebted to my husband for his support and with his technical help in displaying photographs.

Edna Hunneysett

Early Autumn 1951

Emma snuggled under her blankets, curled up with her knees bent, a letter in one hand and a tiny, slimline, black torch in the other. Lights were out in the junior dormitory and she didn't want anyone catching her reading. Hence the need to appear to be asleep under the covers. As far as she was aware, when the lights were out, it meant exactly that. She didn't want to be reported for breaking the rules. She was still trying to remember all the rules since arriving in September. It was now well into October with half-term two weeks away when the boarders go back home to their families, but only for a very short visit from Friday to Tuesday. She could hardly wait. She quietly slid the pages from the envelope, the glow from the torch revealing neat, squarish writing, not like her own slanty scrawl, she thought. Emma began reading, pushing her straight, short-cut, black hair from her eyes, as she'd removed the hairclip normally keeping it in place, when getting into bed.

This was the first letter from her older sister Martha, aged twelve, since this new beginning at boarding school. Having previously skimmed the letter, when seated at a table in the boarders' room doing her homework in silence as always, she wanted to read it again slowly and relish every word. She was so happy at receiving Martha's letter filled with lots of news, different from her mother's in her weekly, short letter to her daughter. Emma missed Martha, but meeting with Faith, another new boarder, eased the ache inside her as Faith was kind to her. As she began reading, her mind drifted back to that very first day when she'd arrived, nervous and shy and wondering what it would be like at the convent boarding grammar school.

'I'll have to go now, Emma, or we'll miss the next bus. I'll write soon.' Mary, her deep brown, teary eyes, over-shadowed by her long, black lashes, normally a vivacious, attractive woman with her mop of curly, short, black hair, was today very downcast, struggling to leave her daughter, knowing she wouldn't see her until half-term in seven weeks. Mary and Emma's dad, Tom, thought it a good decision to accept a place for Emma, the third of their six children, as a boarder at the convent grammar school after she'd passed her eleven plus exam. They envisaged that this would give her a better opportunity to study than being at home, as conditions on the family's isolated rented farm on the North Yorkshire moors were not ideal. They realised this after their eldest child, Tim, who passed his eleven plus exam two years earlier, began travelling daily the ten miles plus into Whitby to attend a grammar school there and on returning to the farmhouse each evening, explained to his parents that

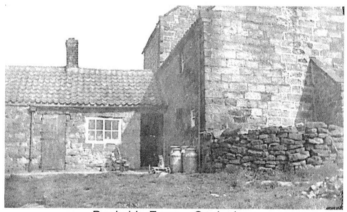

Bankside Farm – Coals door

he needed space to do his homework. In their overcrowded farmhouse kitchen cum living room, finding space for him to spread out his exercise and textbooks was very difficult.

Mary and Tom hadn't the income to pay for their daughter's education at a boarding school, but when Emma passed her eleven plus exam, the local county council offered her a choice of grammar schools including the boarding school, the fees funded by the authority under the means-tested system. She was very excited at the time even though it meant leaving not only Tim and Martha but also her three younger siblings. Her mother told the nuns, when Tom and Mary took Emma for her interview in August, that she felt it would be to their daughter's advantage to study under the supervised conditions that the convent offered, rather than her struggling to find space for study in their kitchen amidst the distractions of chatter and goings-on of family life, including the cooking and cleaning.

At the time, Emma was delighted at the prospect of a boarding school, as details of such places sounded very exciting in a fictional story book she'd read.
'And are you sure you want to go?' Mary asked, when plans were first discussed.
'Oh, yes,' said Emma, with great enthusiasm. 'I'll love it.' She could barely imagine the life compared with the present one where they took candles to bed and Tilley oil-filled lamps were their means of light downstairs. 'Fancy being able to put a switch down on the wall and lights come on,' she mused. That's what she'd read. 'There will be toilets where you pulled a chain and water flushed them out, not like our bucket in the outdoor lavatory with a wooden board for a seat and which dad emptied when it was full. Proper toilet paper too instead of the hard, shiny pieces they used, torn

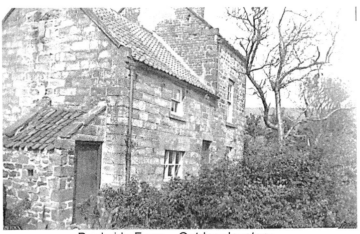

Bankside Farm – Outdoor lavatory

from The Farmers Weekly that lay in the corner in the dust among cobwebs, dead flies and stray, live spiders that crawled from their webs and needed swiping off the seat. I bet there aren't black beetles scuttling around in their toilets.' Her enthusiasm was unrelenting whilst waiting for her adventure to begin.

When the big day arrived, Emma, with Mary, travelled the thirty miles or so by bus to Scarborough leaving Martha, now a responsible twelve-year-old, in charge of the younger siblings, with Tom around. He'd taken a short time out to chauffeur Mary, sitting beside him on the David Brown tractor's double seat and with Emma in the link-box attachment at the back, holding her two cases, to the bus stop on the main road. Apart from the horse and cart, the tractor, that Tom recently purchased, was the family's only means of transport and regularly used to take them over the mile moor track and another mile on the tarmac road to Windrush village church on Sundays.

The David Brown red tractor with its double seat was ideal for picking up a passenger at the bus stop which Tom managed to occasionally. The family appreciated this mode of transport especially when carrying heavy shopping home over the moor. He'd made the link-box, a wooden contraption to go at the back, specifically to enable some of the children to have a ride on the tractor instead of the two-mile walk when they went to church. The tractor was a common sight in the village as Tom usually parked it alongside the cars on The Green on Sunday mornings. It was known as Moorbeck Express after a local farmer and friend of Tom's told a parishioner that Tom Holmes had gotten himself an Express, Moorbeck being the name of the hamlet wherein their farm was situated. Word soon spread. The name stuck. The children didn't care, as a ride on the tractor was better than the long walk and they would wave to the cars passing them by as they chugged their way on the tarmac road to the village.

Mrs Williams, a motherly, elderly lady with kindly, blue eyes and wispy, grey hair tied in a bun, joined Emma and her mother at the bus stop. She lived on a neighbouring farm not as far down the valley as the Holmes farm and she'd offered to go with Mary on her excursion. She knew that Mary would be alone on the long journey home and may need comfort. After arriving in Scarborough, they'd walked through the streets from the bus station, Mary carrying the large, cumbersome, brown case and Emma clutching a smaller one. The little party stopped several times to ask the way to the convent in Queen Street before finally reaching their destination.

They were now standing in a square-shaped room, having been ushered there by a nun on their arrival. Emma remembered this little nun greeting them when she'd been for her interview because the nun seemed such a jovial person with her twinkling, blue eyes and ready smile even though she wore such weird clothing, Emma remembered thinking. The nun was dressed in black from head to toe, her long robe reaching to her black, laced-up shoes and with a thick headpiece hanging to her shoulders. A white band covered her forehead allowing only her facial features to be seen; not a strand of hair in sight.

Emma took her eyes off the nun and gazed around. 'This must be the cloakroom,' she thought, seeing rows of coat hooks along three sides of the dark green walls and wooden open-ended boxes at floor level, underneath the hooks. It was not unlike the cloakroom at the village school that she'd attended, a school with one classroom and only one teacher most of the time, a school that was a two mile daily walk each way from their farm. 'My goodness,' Emma exclaimed, quietly, just realising that she wouldn't even have to walk outside to go to school. She noticed a heavy-looking closed wooden door in the corner of the smallish room and was wondering where it led to, when the nun's voice broke her thoughts.
'Just wait there, please,' instructed the chubby, smiling nun, pushing her thick-lensed glasses to settle more comfortably onto the bridge of her snub nose. 'I understand that Joanne Raymons will be with you shortly to look after you,' she added, before giving them a beaming smile and disappearing into the corridor.

Whilst they were waiting, Emma, was beginning to look rather forlorn, hunching her shoulders as she was prone to do when nervous, her dark brown eyes welling up with tears. She was suddenly feeling scared, after all the build-up and excitement thinking about her new school, but it was hitting home now that she wouldn't have her sister around. She could always voice her anxieties to Martha especially when

11

daily walking together the two miles to school, but Martha, not having passed the second half of the eleven plus exam, remained at the village school. Emma was on her own now and the realisation of the enormity of what was happening was dawning.

'We'll have to go now Emma, otherwise we'll miss our bus. Joanne will be with you any minute now,' Mary said. Emma gave her mother one last hug before reaching for her hankie from her coat pocket. She was fighting back the tears whilst waiting for her mother to leave. She recalled Mary raising a half smile as she gazed at her daughter for the last time. With Mrs Williams leading the way, Mary turned her back on Emma and walked out of the room, down the corridor and though the large, wooden doors onto the street without glancing back, feeling very sorrowful. Basically, the only life Emma knew was Bankside farm and walking to school with her siblings and going to church on Sundays. Mary wondered how her little girl would cope. Had they made the right decision? Would Emma be looked after properly and who would comfort her when things went wrong? Such thoughts buzzed round in Mary's head as she walked with Mrs Williams through the streets of Scarborough.

Left inside the convent alone, Emma was struggling to see through her blurred, tearful eyes. Suddenly it didn't seem quite so exciting, this boarding school idea. She felt abandoned, with a big lump in her throat and a pain in the pit of her tummy.

'Hello. You must be Emma. I've been looking out for you.' Standing in front of Emma was a tall, slim girl with long, blond hair hanging loosely round her shoulders. 'I'm Joanne and my mother visited your home in the summer holidays which was when your mam asked if I would help you settle in.' Joanne, from another village on the Yorkshire moors, with no pangs of homesickness and well used to the boarding school regime, was beginning her lower fifth year. She'd arrived earlier and taken her cases to the dormitory, leaving her mother, who'd made the journey with her, engrossed in a conversation with one of the nuns on teaching methods. After returning to say goodbye to her mother and being told that Emma had arrived, Joanne went to find her.

Many weeks earlier, word spread around the villages close to Windrush that Emma was going to the convent boarding school and the news reached Mrs Raymons, the mother of Joanne. Mrs Raymons was a supply teacher for the local village schools in the area and was aware of the Holmes family through occasionally teaching at Windrush village Catholic school. On learning about Emma, Mrs Raymons, an older version of her tall, blond-haired daughter, had given some thought as to how she might help as she knew the Holmes had very little money and struggled with their large family. It was in August that she visited the family, making a journey on the local Moordale bus and walking the last mile or so across the moorland track to Bankside farm. Before going, she sorted through items of school clothing that Joanne had grown out of and took some with her on her visit.

'It's the uniform they wear,' she explained to Mary. 'The dress is a bit faded but should do.'

'I suppose it will be all right,' thought Mary, dubiously.

'The dark brown coat is in good condition except for a patch on the pocket,' continued Mrs Raymons, a well-dressed woman and today looking very smart even in her casual, grey trousers and summer jacket to match, but always with a kindly disposition. 'Our Joanne left some biscuits in the pocket and a mouse nibbled its way in. Shouldn't be noticed much, though.'

Mary was very grateful as uniform costs were not covered by the county council grant and she was aware of just how expensive it was to purchase the necessary items from the list she'd received. The coat was on the large size for Emma.

'She will grow into it,' commented Mrs Raymons. 'Our Joanne is quite a big girl.'

'You'll ask Joanne to look out for Emma at school, won't you? She's a bit shy and nervous,' Mary requested, fretting about her daughter.

'Yes, I will. Our Joanne will keep an eye on her until she settles down. Don't you worry about that.' On returning home, Mrs Raymons explained to Joanne how anxious Emma's mother was at the thought of their daughter starting boarding school and Joanne reassured her mother that she would try to help Emma the first few days, in case of problems.

'I don't suppose that I'll see much of her, though, Mam,' Joanne volunteered, 'as our form rooms are in a different part of the school to the new starters. I'll do my best though.'

Now back at school, Joanne was remembering her mother's words and tried to reassure Emma.

'You'll be fine, you know,' she continued. 'Come on. Take off your coat and hat and hang them on the hook under your name and I'll show you where to go. Those open wooden boxes, below where we hang our coats, are for our outdoor shoes.' Emma remembered from the list of essential purchases that it was requisite for each boarder to have two pairs of shoes. 'We change into our outdoor shoes each day for the walk after classes,' Joanne continued. 'Otherwise wear your indoor shoes. By the way, although this looks like a cloakroom, it's called a vestry. Just so you know if anyone uses that word. We wait in here each evening after supper before we go into chapel for night prayers, through that door there, see?' she explained, pointing to the wooden door in the corner. 'It's the same for morning prayers or Mass and you must wear your hat in chapel, just like you would in church back home. We normally don't talk in here either. Okay?' Emma nodded and dried her eyes whilst hoping that she would be able to remember all these details.

'Thank you,' she whispered.

'Just ask me if you're worried about anything,' Joanne added, reassuringly.

Emma was finding it difficult to carry the large, fully expanded, brown suitcase in one hand as she couldn't change hands with already having a much smaller case in the other. Mary had painstakingly selected the most necessary items needed from the original list of suggested clothing and these did not take up much space, but the bedding was bulkier; hence the cumbersome suitcase.

'It's not as if I can put her old clothes in. She hasn't much decent to wear,' she'd said to Tom, her husband, when packing the cases. 'Apparently they change out of their uniform each evening into their own clothes. I've packed her best skirt and a couple of jumpers. I hope they'll do.' Tom nodded. He'd come into the farmhouse from his work to see how things were progressing. It was then he'd offered to take Mary with Emma on the tractor to the tarmac road where they were to catch the bus, as it was a tedious walk with the heavy case.

'There's still enough clothes and stuff in them to make them feel weighty even though mam said that she'd cut the list right down,' thought Emma, as she struggled along with her cases, trailing behind Joanne.
'I'll carry that,' Joanne offered, taking Emma's very large case, as she saw that Emma was lagging. Joanne led the way along the broad corridor, with its shiny, polished floor. 'That's the refectory,' she pointed out, indicating the double wooden doors on the right. It's where we have our meals.'
'Strange word, that,' thought Emma. 'We eat in a kitchen,' she informed Joanne. 'We don't have a separate room.' She hadn't heard of a refectory before and was trying to memorise another new word.

Joanne continued with information.
'Normally we wouldn't be allowed to talk in this corridor either but today is an exception to the rule.' At the end of the corridor, Joanne turned right and began climbing the first flight of stairs, nodding and smiling at other boarders, who were either wandering down empty handed or lugging cases up the stairs.
'A new one, is she?' questioned a tall girl with a round, freckled face and her ginger hair tied back in a ponytail. 'You'll have to get those locks tied back for tomorrow,' she added, cheekily, to Joanne. Joanne laughed.
'Yes, I will, and yes, she is,' she replied. 'This is Emma who comes from one of the villages near where I live. I'm just showing her the ropes. This is Margaret, now beginning her second year here and not a care in the world. Have you had a good holiday?' Margaret nodded.
'Don't worry,' she said to Emma. 'You'll soon get used to it. I know what I felt like last year.' She seemed to Emma to be a bubbly, outgoing character, confidently engaging with other

girls on the staircase, as she struggled with her own case, a step or two ahead of Joanne.

Emma followed Joanne, taking the stairs around a bend and up another flight to the first floor, where a long corridor led off to the left.

'Another two flights, yet,' said Joanne. They stopped and put the cases down momentarily, to rest. 'That's the boarders' room,' she pointed out, helpfully, indicating a door to the left, off the corridor. 'The small room opposite is Mother Monica's office. She's the headmistress of the school as well as overseeing the boarders. You'll meet her in a minute. Those are two toilets there on the right near her office. I don't know if you noticed but there were two at the end of the corridor downstairs directly under those two.' Emma wondered why they called a nun, Mother, but was too timid to ask. They picked up the cases and turned to go up the next flight of stairs, Joanne acknowledging a handful of girls coming down. 'Do you think you might have a cubicle this year, Margaret?' Joanne questioned, as Margaret paused on the next step.

'I hope so. I don't fancy another year in the junior dorm.'

'Will I ever get to know all these faces?' Emma wondered. 'Will I even remember which way to go, which corridor to turn into?' Up the next flight they went, pausing halfway as they turned the corner.

They finally reached the top of the fourth flight of stairs and stopped outside the dormitory door where a nun was in conversation with another young lady. The girls waited for her to finish. Emma studied the nun, tall, thin and elderly with thin-rimmed glasses perched on her nose and wearing a black, full-length, long-sleeved, plain dress of a heavy material.

'Just like they wore when I came for my interview,' thought Emma. The nun's hands were tucked under a narrow, blue piece of material reaching from her neckband to her black, lace-up shoes, like a long scarf. Black headgear rested on her shoulders with the same white band on her forehead as the other nun. Emma was mesmerised by the clothing, just as she'd been on that earlier visit. She'd never seen anyone dressed like this. She also noticed this time, a long string of

16

rosary beads, large, wooden and black with a crucifix at the end, hanging down one side of the dress. Emma's rosary beads were tiny in comparison and she kept them in a little plastic box. Emma thought that the nun looked quite severe, not like the chubby, smiling nun, who opened the door for them. Emma remembered that the little nun was all in black, but they'd addressed her as Sister. She pondered about this. Then she recalled that the other nun didn't have the blue piece of cloth hanging down the front. 'Maybe, that's the clue,' she thought. 'The ones with the extra blue piece are addressed as Mother and the ones just in black as Sister. Maybe it's to do with whatever job they do. I'll ask someone later.'

'Mother Monica, this is Emma Holmes, one of the new girls,' said Joanne.
'Hello, Emma,' Mother Monica greeted her, with a half-smile. 'Take Emma down to the junior dormitory, please, will you, Joanne. You have a cubicle on the garden side. Hello, Margaret. You have a cubicle this year, down the street side.' She turned away to greet another newcomer.
Joanne, Emma and Margaret walked into the main dormitory. Narrow corridors led off to right and left. A broad corridor lay down the centre, flanked on either side by white-curtained cubicles.
'My cubicle is to the right and around the corner,' explained Joanne. 'It's called the garden side because cubicles down that side overlook the convent grounds. I'll take you to your dormitory. There's no talking in the dormitories, by the way. You must ask permission from the nun in charge if you want to speak to anyone. She sits at that small table, there.'
Joanne pointed to a wooden square table situated in the centre corridor. There was a hand bell on it.
'I wonder what that's for,' Emma mused.

Margaret led the way along the short corridor on the left, followed by Joanne, still heaving Emma's large case. They turned down another narrow corridor with windows on the left over-looking the street and cubicles on the right. The white curtains were closed across some of the cubicles. Other curtains were pulled back to reveal a bed and locker, a small wardrobe and a washbasin. Margaret was looking for her name.

'I'm here,' she said. 'I'm so pleased I've got a cubicle. I'll see you later.' She walked into one about halfway down the corridor and placing her case on the bed, drew her curtain. At the far end of the corridor was a door. As Joanne approached it, she indicated to Emma, the last cubicle. 'That's the head boarder's cubicle. She's there to keep an eye on the junior dormitory which is where you are sleeping. Any noise and she'll be in to tell you off.'

Joanne opened the door and they walked inside. Emma gazed around. The dormitory was full of narrow beds, five down one side and six down the other. They were in neat rows and beside each bed was a locker. At the far end of the room was a row of five white porcelain washbasins. The two girls walked down the dormitory until they found Emma's name above an empty bed, fourth from the end on the left-hand side.

'Unpack and make your bed,' said Joanne, indicating the empty bed. 'You have your own locker. Any clothes that you need to hang up, go in the large wardrobe over there,' she explained, pointing to the wardrobe to the right of the door through which they'd entered. 'You all share that wardrobe. I'll see you later. When you've finished unpacking, you need to take your suitcases to the attic where we store them, but I think Mother Monica will be showing you where to go. Then you'll probably be brought down to the boarders' room. I'll be in there. Okay?' Emma nodded, feeling very apprehensive again. With these instructions, Joanne smiled and walked out, leaving Emma standing by her unmade bed.

Emma glanced round, nervously. A couple of girls were unpacking their cases. Another was sitting on her bed, having finished making it. Others were covering their blankets with fancy bedspreads or embroidered eiderdowns, topped with elegantly stitched, cloth cases, which she assumed were for pyjamas. One or two beds displayed only a mattress, an uncovered pillow and clean, white sheets and pillowcase. Emma opened her large suitcase and took out two plain blankets and a plain pink eiderdown. She laid them to one side whilst she emptied the cases of her few possessions and put them away in her locker. Putting the cases by her bed, she set to and made it up with the crisp, white sheets and after putting a cover on the pillow, pushed a pair of pyjamas under it. Another two girls arrived in the dormitory and busied themselves with bed making and emptying suitcases. They mostly looked scared and bewildered and slightly lost. There was a little whispering going on and a lot of furtive glances.

'Have you managed everything?' enquired a gentle voice behind her. Emma turned around to face a slightly taller girl than herself and a little broader too, with wavy, thick, auburn hair cascading round her smiling face.
'I'm Faith, and I'm new too. I guess you are. You must be Emma,' she added, reading the name above the bed. 'I'm feeling a bit lost. I thought I'd say hello.'
'I think I've done everything. I'm a bit nervous, though.' Faith nodded but said no more as the door opened and Mother Monica walked in. She stood and waited until there was complete silence in the room.

'Bring your empty cases and follow me, please,' she instructed. The girls trooped out and followed the nun through to the dormitory's main entrance where she pointed out a flight of steep, small wooden stairs with a single light bulb at the top. 'Just follow the older girls to the attic rooms and leave your suitcases there.' It was a tight squeeze with their bulky cases when passing boarders descended the stairs. The attic rooms were dark and eerie, lit only by the occasional bare light bulb. In one corner was a stack of cases. Some wire ran along under the rafters as if for clothes to be aired there. After depositing their cases, the other girls went back down the wooden stairs, with Emma trailing, thinking that she wouldn't like to go up there alone. She thought it was spooky.

'Would you mind taking these new girls down to the boarders' room please and show them their lockers?' requested Mother Monica to Margaret, as she appeared at the bottom of the wooden stairs. Margaret nodded.
'Come on, Emma,' she said, remembering her name and with the other girls listening, 'I'll show you.' Following Margaret, Emma now noticed that the stairs were nothing

like hers at home even though she'd already walked up them. The steps were quite shallow but twice as long in width and deeper in breadth than the little, wooden ones that she was used to. They seemed to her to be made of shiny, mottled marble. The group of girls walked carefully down them. There were older boarders already walking down the stairs, two or three abreast and chattering like magpies.
'In silence, please, and single file. There is no talking on the stairs at any time,' Mother Monica called after them. The girls obediently moved into a single line and no more words were spoken. Emma remembered what Joanne told her about silence in the corridors and it seemed to her that everywhere they went, it was no talking. She was wondering when they could talk.

The boarders' room was long and narrow and filled with tables and chairs, six chairs approximately to a table. There were many windows along one wall, that overlooked Queen Street and along this wall at the centre was a table with a small hand bell on it and one chair behind it.
'Another bell, just like in the dormitory,' Emma thought, gazing around the room and trying to take things in. On the opposite wall was a stack of small lockers, each with a pupil's name on.

'We come here in the evening after we've been on a walk and then changed out of our uniforms and had tea,' Margaret explained to the group of new girls standing around her. 'You'll soon learn by watching what the others do. We do our homework in here in silence. That table is for the nun to sit at as we are always supervised. If you need to go to the toilet or speak to another person about homework, you approach the desk and ask the supervising nun for permission. She rings the bell when it's time to put our homework books away, but you'll see what happens. So, don't worry.' There were girls standing around, talking and laughing.
'Joanne. Hello,' called one of the girls loudly, across the room. Emma glanced across and saw Joanne smiling broadly.
'You'll find your name on a locker,' Margaret continued to the listening new starters, pointing the lockers out for them. 'I'm

just going to speak to some friends.' Soon there was a group around her, giggling and chattering, catching up on holiday news. This was replicated around the room except for the new boarders. They were easy to pick out, standing or sitting and gazing tentatively around, looking lonely and anxious.

Emma, unable to see Faith anywhere, was walking over to find her name on one of the lockers when she was approached by an older, heavily built girl with short, dark, curly hair, pencil-thin eyebrows and a snub nose.
'What's your name then?' she questioned, in quite an authoritative voice, Emma thought.
'Emma Holmes.'
'Where do you live?'
'At Bankside farm.'
'Where's that?'
'In Moorbeck.'
'Yes, but where is it?' the questioning continued.
'It's two miles from Windrush, you know, over t' moors,' explained Emma.
'Oh! You're a little woolly-back, then,' the girl responded, rather sarcastically. She smiled. 'And do you like the idea of boarding school?'
'Well, I've read about them in books and they sounded exciting. I thought I'd like it,' Emma replied, timidly, feeling a bit bombarded, and beginning to think maybe it isn't so good after all.

This conversation was cut short by the sound of hands clapping. Emma looked across the room to see Mother Monica standing in the doorway. Silence descended. The seated boarders stood up, with new ones among them slightly slower at getting up than the others. The pointers of the round wall-mounted white clock at the far end of the room, with its large, black numbering, gave the time as twenty minutes past seven.
'Good evening, girls,' said Mother Monica.
'Good evening, Mother,' they chorused.
'Form a line and go down for supper, please. In silence,' she reminded them, standing back to allow the girls to stream past her. Emma sidled into the line as the girls left the boarders' room. They went down the stairs, lining up along

the bottom corridor in single file, with the leading girl coming to a halt outside the refectory door. Emma wondered what happened next. Mother Monica was walking past the silent queue, making her way to the head of the line, whereupon she opened the refectory door and went inside. The girls followed slowly, entering a long, airy room that displayed several large windows looking out onto Queen Street.

Inside the refectory were tables and chairs placed at intervals, far more than were required for the forty or so boarders. The girls crowded forward to inspect a plan of the seating arrangements pinned onto a notice board on the side wall opposite the windows. Emma was feeling quite numb inside, bewildered and worried. It was all so different. She hung back until many of the girls, having found their allocated places, moved away from the notice. After studying the plan, she moved across to the third table under the windows, noticing that others were not sitting down but were standing behind their chairs. She did likewise. Her position was at the bottom end of the table and she recognised that one of the girls standing at their table was the same girl who asked her all the questions. This worried Emma a little. There were two girls to each side and one at the top of the table. She was hoping that maybe Faith would be on the same table, but no such luck.

After grace was said by Mother Monica, there was a scraping and scuffling as the boarders pulled out their chairs and sat down. Sitting down on a hard, brown, wooden chair reminded Emma of home and tears welled up. She blinked, swallowed and hung her head whilst she fought to regain control. She didn't want anyone to see how homesick she was. Three of the girls removed their serviettes from the serviette rings, that they'd brought to the table, placing the serviettes on their knees, the rings remaining on the table. Emma watched. She'd never seen serviettes used before.
'I'm Judith, and you are?' the girl at the top of the table, sitting opposite Emma, asked. Her light brown hair was cut short in a fringe almost covering her eyebrows. Her eyes were steely blue.
'Emma Holmes,' Emma whispered, hoping no-one noticed her wiping a tear from her eye.

'Have you brought your serviette and ring?' Emma shook her head.

'They're in my locker in the bedroom.'

'Well, bring them down to breakfast in the morning, please. That goes for anyone else who has forgotten,' Judith added, looking around the table. 'We keep them in this drawer here after each meal,' she explained, demonstrating by pulling out a small drawer from under the table and then closing it. 'By the way, it's a dormitory, here, not a bedroom,' she added, kindly, smiling at Emma. Emma nodded. Only now did she realise that some of the boarders were carrying their serviettes with them as they'd walked into the refectory. 'So much to take in,' she thought. The other girls were chattering.

'I know you know each other but can you tell Emma your names, please,' Judith requested. They obliged.

Supper began, consisting of bread and cheese and stewed plums. The mealtime ended with the sound of a bell. Mother Monica was bringing the girls to silence.

'Another bell, the third bell I've seen already,' thought Emma. 'In the dormitory, on the table in the boarders' room and here, but now I know why there are little bells, because they make us stop talking,' she decided. The girls rose from their seats and after placing their chairs correctly at the tables, stood to attention.

'After thanksgiving grace, we will go to the vestry ready for night prayers in chapel, as we do each evening,' instructed Mother Monica, with her eyes glancing at the new boarders. 'Don't forget that we walk in silence down the corridor and no talking in the vestry either.'

On arriving in the vestry, the girls were pushing around, retrieving their brown hats from the pegs and pulling them onto their heads. Emma felt someone taking her arm.

'We need to join the young ones at the front,' whispered Faith. 'Maureen has just told me.'

'Who is Maureen?' questioned Emma, very quietly, aware they weren't meant to be talking.

'She is the head boarder. She's very nice. Come on.'

Together they made their way to near the front of the queue. Someone opened the chapel door and the stream of girls

walked quietly in pairs into the chapel.
On entering the chapel, Emma gazed around whilst following
the pair ahead walking down the centre aisle to the front.

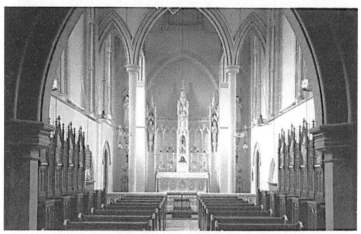

The Convent Chapel

The benches at each side were quite small with space for
only four or five persons. Narrow side aisles separated the
benches from large single pews, some occupied by nuns
silently praying. Carvings of Christ's journey on the way to
be crucified, known as The Stations of the Cross, were
displayed around the walls.
'They're not like ours at St Peter's in Windrush,' she thought,
remembering the church in the village where the Holmes
family attended Mass each Sunday. 'These are much
smaller but beautifully carved.' She gazed up at the altar
where a small crucifix took centre place above the
tabernacle. She brought her mind back to the present.

Someone was leading prayers out loud with a chorus of
voices responding. Although preoccupied with taking in her
surroundings and not really concentrating, Emma
automatically joined in the *Our Father*. Another girl started
the hymn and others sang with her which was when Emma
realised there were books at the end of each bench, prayer
books and hymn books. The singing ceased and she felt
someone nudging her and realised she needed to move.

The girls were leaving their seats and standing up. Most of the girls genuflected when leaving their bench but one or two new ones gave a sort of dip with the knee as if they weren't sure how to genuflect. 'Maybe they don't go to church,' mused Emma. She followed the girls filing out in the same orderly fashion as when they came in, removing their hats immediately they stepped from the chapel.

'In single file, please, with no talking, to the main hall for recreation,' voiced Mother Monica. Emma was exceedingly tired. The days of build-up and excitement finishing with these extremely exhausting last few hours were taking their toll on her. How she longed for her bed.

Meekly, Emma followed the girls down the long corridor, through the doors at the end, turning right and walking along another corridor with its well-polished, wooden floors and flanked on one side with rooms, until finally arriving in a large hall. She noticed a stage at one end of the hall with very long, dark red curtains pulled well back. Then she gazed at long, wooden bars across the length of one wall and a single door in the corner at the back wall. On the opposite side to the wooden bars, were large, glass windows with a set of exit doors in the centre. She was intrigued as she had no idea what the wooden bars were for. The girls broke rank and milled around talking and laughing. Emma spied Joanne surrounded by other girls, all chattering noisily. She walked across and stood hesitantly on the edge of the group.

'This is Emma Holmes,' said Joanne, 'and I've been asked to help her settle in. This is the assembly hall and it's also where the indoor physical exercise classes are held, known as PE,' she explained to Emma. The girls smiled briefly before continuing their conversation which seemed to be mainly about boys, but Emma wasn't interested in boys. After standing around for a little on the edge of Joanne's friendly circle, Emma became bored and felt like an eavesdropper and a bit of a nuisance.

'As kind as she is, I don't think Joanne wants me hanging around,' she thought, realising that Joanne probably would rather Emma went elsewhere. She spotted Faith who was walking towards her and they moved away. 'I'm very tired,' volunteered Emma, thinking of something to say.

'Come and meet Audrey,' invited Faith. 'She's new, too. I've just discovered that she comes from Bartown, the small, market town where I come from, except that she lives in a different part of it. She lives in the posh part but don't tell her I said that. We go to the same picture house though as there is only one in Bartown. I go a lot to the pictures with my mam as we are not too far from it and can walk there.'

'Fancy living near a picture house,' Emma thought.

She remembered once going to Whitby on the bus with her mam and sitting on unusual chairs in a darkened, very large room with a massive screen and pictures flashing across it. That was the only time she'd ever been to one. As they sauntered across the hall, she noticed two or three girls quietly reading. 'That's what I'll do,' she decided. 'I'll get hold of a book somehow and then next time I'll be able to read in a quiet corner.' She voiced her thoughts to Faith.

'I think I saw Audrey unpacking some when we were emptying our cases. She might lend you one,' Faith suggested. 'I'll mention it to her, if you like.' Faith introduced Emma to Audrey. The minutes ticked slowly by as Audrey, a tall, slim girl, her blond hair in two long plaits, chatted to Faith.

'We were just catching up on some of the places we know with living in the same place,' voiced Faith, as Audrey moved away to speak to another boarder.

'I noticed Audrey was one of the girls who didn't genuflect in church, I mean chapel,' commented Emma, in her effort to make conversation, after Audrey was out of earshot.

'Well that's because she's probably not a Catholic,' replied Faith. 'I've not seen her when I go to church with my mam and there's only one Catholic church in our town.'

'I didn't realise they weren't all Catholics. It must be quite hard for them having to go to chapel as often as we'll have to.'

'Well, I suppose they're aware of this when they decide to come here. I think there are some boarders who aren't Catholic, but my mam told me that the nuns take in some who have difficulties at home or some other reason,' Faith explained. 'I don't think that's the case with Audrey, though. Apparently, her parents own a shop and they live above it.

Maybe it would be too busy for her to get her homework done. Anyway, why did you come?'

Emma gave this some thought.
'I suppose mam and dad wanted me to come after I'd passed my eleven plus and this school was on a list of five Catholic grammar schools to choose from. There isn't a Catholic one at Whitby, our nearest town, ten miles or so away from the farm. My brother, Tim, who's two years older than me, goes to the grammar school in Whitby but he doesn't like it much. He gets teased a lot by the town lads 'cos we're a bit different, I suppose. Martha is a year older than me, but she didn't pass and she's still at the little village school in Windrush. Our home is messy and there isn't much room as there are three more, younger than me. Tim already struggles to find space to do his homework. I think they thought that I'd be able to have more space and be able to concentrate better here.'
'But it's expensive this place,' replied Faith. 'Are you well off?'
'No. The Council pay the fees. We were means-tested if you know what that means. My mam explained to me about means-testing. They check your money coming in and what you need to live on, depending on how many are in your family. We only rent our farm and we never have any spare money. I know my mam is always waiting for the milk cheque every month as that's where our money comes from. Sometimes it's not as much as they think it will be and she worries. It's up and down depending on how much milk the cows give. She did have to buy my bedding and uniform though, but Joanne's mam gave me a dress and coat that Joanne has outgrown. Do you come from a big family?'

Faith was wondering about how much she should tell Emma about her home life when Mother Monica, who was supervising them, stood up and clapped her hands.
'I'll tell you some other time,' she replied, whilst glancing at the clock on the far wall. The pointers showed that it was twenty minutes past eight o'clock. Again, for the umpteenth time it seemed to Emma, the girls were lining up in silence. Then the long walk back along the corridors and up the flights of stairs to the dormitory.

'No more conversation now 'til morning,' Emma thought, as she made her way silently behind others, although there was some whispering between the girls, she noticed, if they were far enough away from the nun. 'I wish I was going to bed with Martha as we always have a good chat in bed but very quietly or mam or dad shout upstairs to tell us to be quiet, in case we wake up the little ones. It's lovely having a sister only a year older,' she mused. 'Maybe she'll write if she's not too busy helping dad with the milking and such like.' Emma was beginning to feel weepy again but on arriving at the dormitory door, she was distracted.

Although Emma knew about electric lights, she still found it fascinating to see the lights come on at the touch of a switch. At home, they carried candles or torches when going to the outside toilet or upstairs to bed. Electricity was new to her. She was one of the first into the junior dormitory and found the switch herself, just inside the door. She smiled as she watched the lights flick on.

The dormitory was soon filled with young girls, mostly rather nervous new ones.
'After stripping to your vest and knickers, you must wash before putting on your nightwear and no sleeping in your vests,' voiced Mother Monica, on arriving in the junior dormitory. 'Are you listening, Susanna?' she asked of the girl with her back to the nun and whispering to another girl. Susanna, on hearing her name, turned around.
Yes, Mother,' she replied. Susanna was short and plump, with thick, black hair hanging down her back to her waist.
'You know the rules, Susanna, this being your second year. Make sure that your hair is plaited in the morning. If it's not Mother Teresa on duty, it will be Sister Dorothy who will help if you need assistance. She recently joined our community here and will sometimes replace Mother Teresa in the dormitory.' Susanna nodded. 'Two to a basin, but three to the end one. That will be Susanna, Polly and Emma,' continued Mother Monica, 'and lights out at nine o'clock.' With that, she turned on her heel and disappeared through the door, closing it after herself. Emma sensed a sigh of relief in the room.

'We'll take turns on who goes first,' said Susanna, walking towards Emma, having glanced at the name above her bed. She was rather bossy in her attitude and full of confidence. 'I'll go first tonight and in the morning. You follow me, Polly,' she instructed to another girl standing opposite them, having learnt her name earlier, 'which means you'll be last this time, Emma. Okay?' The two girls nodded, unwilling to argue with Susanna. Emma said *hello* to Polly whilst noticing her cropped, brown hair. Polly nodded offhandedly and returned to her bedside.

Whilst waiting for a turn at the washbasin, Emma undressed and put on her dressing gown, before sitting sat down on her bed to wait. She'd never owned a dressing gown before. It was pink and very long, soft and cosy. Her slippers were new as well and trimmed with pink fur. As she put them on, she was reminded of her mam and home and felt a wave of tears surging up, but she blinked a few times. She couldn't let all these girls see her crying. Emma was one of the last into bed. She was wearing her brand-new pyjamas, floral patterned and made of winceyette for extra warmth. She was tired out. She heard someone come into the dormitory and say a short prayer and then the lights went out. Within minutes, Emma was fast asleep. Even the traffic on the street below outside their windows failed to disturb her, on this, her first night away from Bankside farm.

****

Emma jerked and came to, realising, after recalling that first traumatic day, that she'd been here for five weeks now. It seemed an age. It was reading Martha's letter that triggered off the reminiscing of the events of that first day, but Emma wasn't aware of her mam's reaction on leaving her in the vestry. After Mary and her neighbour walked out of the convent, her tears flowed. They walked quickly through the streets to the bus station, having to ask directions just once, eager to keep to their schedule as the buses ran infrequently. It was a tedious journey home via Whitby and along the moor road towards Middlesbrough. A few miles out of Whitby, they alighted to walk the remaining mile over the rough cart track to Moorbeck, Tom having already informed his wife earlier that he wouldn't be able to pick her up at the bus stop.

'But you'll manage as you'll have nothing to carry,' he'd added. It wasn't a problem for Mary. She'd walked the track many a time when knowing how busy Tom was.

'Thank you so much for coming with us today,' Mary said to her neighbour, as they parted company. Mrs Williams lived on the farm halfway into Moorbeck and was taking a different track to reach it. 'It would have been much harder on my own. I'm so grateful.' Mrs Williams smiled. She'd had her own hardships in life, bringing up her children and managing the farm after the death of her husband. She was pleased to help where she could, having known Mary, a town lass, for a while now, struggling over the years with farm life and stark living conditions alongside the demands of a brood of little ones. It was good, she thought, that she generally seemed happier these days. When Mary was in hospital for minor surgery, Mrs Williams had given Tom a few hours help, baking and sorting out the washing. She remembered the tiredness, coping with little ones and helping on the farm, when her children were younger. 'Now, don't you be fretting too much,' Mrs Williams advised. 'That little lass will do fine.' She turned in the direction of her farmhouse alongside the well-worn track and Mary continued down into the valley to Bankside farm, sombre and weary.

'She looked so small and pathetic, Tom, standing there beside her case,' Mary said to her husband, much later in the evening after the younger children were in bed. They were enjoying a late-night woodbine whilst pondering over their decision, made a couple of months ago, to send their daughter to boarding school. 'I thought about it a lot on the bus journey home. I wonder if we've done the right thing sending her away so young. Do you think she'll manage at boarding school at her age with coming from such a rural background? I hope she doesn't get teased about her broad Yorkshire accent. I told that nun that we'd discuss their advice about her having a few elocution lessons. We'd have to pay, though. The grant doesn't cover extras like that. It would be worth it, I think.'
'We did what we thought was best for her, sending her

there,' Tom replied, reassuringly. 'She'll have more opportunities in life getting a good education. Well, that's my opinion anyway and she'd have a difficult job getting her homework done here with three younger bairns around. It's hard enough for Tim when getting back from school at Whitby doing his homework, with the noise and clutter, but this is how it is, you know. When Tim passed his eleven plus exam two years ago, we decided on the grammar school at Whitby, but it hasn't gone down too well with him. Then Martha didn't quite make it. Now it's Emma. Maybe she'll let us know how she feels about those elocution lessons. We'll find the extra money if needs be.' Mary nodded.
'I know what. I'm going to miss my little helper,' she said. 'She's so good with the little ones and it's like our Martha says, things will be different without her.'
'She's right, there,' replied Tom. 'They've never been separated before, those two little lasses but she'll be home for the holidays. They can write to each other. That nun said at the interview that they write home every weekend. It'll only be a day or two and we'll hear from her. Don't fret, lass. Let's go to bed and see what tomorrow brings.'

Long after Tom was asleep, Mary lay thinking, still seeing little Emma's tearful face when they left her standing alone in that cloakroom. She shed a few silent tears before drifting into an uneasy sleep wondering if her daughter would be okay.

Edna Hunneysett

Autumn 1951

Emma, awakening earlier than usual, was still holding
Martha's letter but the torch was sticking into her.
'I must have fallen asleep,' she thought. She quickly
switched the torch off, hoping that the battery had some use
left in it and reaching out to her bedside locker, quietly put
the torch away. It wasn't quite time to get up. 'I'll just have
another read of the letter,' she thought, laying it on her pillow
whilst propping herself up slightly. 'I never read it properly
with thinking about that first evening and falling asleep. I'm
not first on the wash basin, anyway. Martha's writing's very
neat compared with mine and the letters quite large and
easy to read, like mam's writing,' she mused, as she began
reading...

*Mam and dad have gone out to a domino drive and me and
Tim are babysitting. They let us sometimes now I'm twelve
and Tim being thirteen and a half. He's getting taller, you
know. He's doing his homework as he gets loads from that
school at Whitby. Do you get a lot? I can hear Jacob making
noises. He'll go to sleep eventually. He runs around all over
now but then he'll soon be two. He does take some
watching. He's lovely with his twinkling, brown eyes and a
cheeky, lop-sided grin. I look after him a lot now you're not
here, but I still do jobs with dad, milking and cleaning out,
you know. Amy asks where you are. She's a real tomboy,
always getting into scrapes even though she's only five. She
fell from a tree the other day and has a whacking bruise on
her leg. She likes going to school with me and Mark. He's
not grown much and not very big for eight but quite chubby,
but then he likes his food.*
*Dad took me on the tractor for a ride out when he went to
see Mr Fletcher, you know, the farmer across the valley and
up that steep track. It's great having a double seat on the
David Brown as most tractors just have one. I'm glad dad
bought this make. We have a good chat together. He said
he'll take me to a dance at Windrush some time and teach
me to dance, after I'm thirteen on my next birthday. They
have them in the village hall, you know. Maybe he'll let you
go with me after your twelfth birthday as I'll be there with
you. That'll be fun, won't it? They have dances there every*

month, but you'll only get, in the holidays…

Emma paused. She was remembering how much she was missing Martha. Her mind back tracked to one of the worst times which was that very first morning when she woke up in a strange place, slowly opening her eyes and for a moment wondering where she was. Where was Martha? She couldn't feel her next to her. No noise of mam downstairs. Sometimes Amy came into their bed and snuggled up to Emma, but not this morning. What was happening? Then realization crept in. She was at boarding school.

She remembered glancing over to the bed next to hers, but the girl was still sleeping. Emma could hear the cars and buses trundling down street outside, whereas at home, it might be the cock crowing outside or dad calling the cows to come in for milking. Then there was that bell ringing in the distance, the noise getting much louder as the dormitory door opened. It wasn't Mother Monica. This was a different nun, small, wrinkled and old, ringing the hand bell, vigorously. The other girls in the dormitory were slowly sitting up, rubbing their eyes and then gazing around. They were eyeing each other, waiting for someone to move. Susanna was an old hand at this as she'd been a boarder for the last two years, having come at a younger age than most and attended the kindergarten school in Scarborough before moving to the big school. She was soon in her vest and knickers and at the basin to wash and clean her teeth. There was a little whispering amongst some of the girls even though silence was the rule.

One or two girls made their way out and down the side of the curtained cubicles to go to the toilets just outside the main dormitory. Emma followed as she needed the toilet and she couldn't wash until Susanna and Polly finished. There was a queue outside the two toilets.
'Come on. We'll go downstairs,' voiced an older girl, her fiery red dressing gown wrapped tightly round her. 'There are two more toilets on the next floor down.' Emma and one or two more girls followed her but there was a queue there too. Eventually it was her turn. She was fascinated by these toilets, unlike their one toilet at home, which was in a

draughty, small brick building attached to the farmhouse. The children were encouraged to pee outside, around the back of the farmhouse, over a grating so that the bucket didn't fill up as quickly, thus saving Tom having to empty it as often. Martha and Emma, as they got older, preferred to find a more private place to squat, such as around the back of the pigsty.

'Not like this,' Emma thought, pulling the chain and watching the water flush the toilet. 'This is amazing.'

She made her way back to the junior dormitory. Polly was still at the basin and Emma sat on her bed anxiously waiting. She found it embarrassing watching these strangers washing and dressing.

'What if I'm late for breakfast,' she thought. 'I wonder if there is a punishment.' Waves of homesickness washed over her. She gulped to stop the tears.

'Your turn now,' said Polly. 'I'm sorry I kept you waiting so long but Susanna was slow. I'll try and hurry her along tomorrow.' Polly, quietly spoken but with what Emma thought of as a posh, speaking voice, was very polite and courteous.

'Maybe she's a bit shy and not stand-offish like I first thought,' mused Emma. She nodded her thanks and hurriedly went through the washing ritual before speedily dressing. She was almost the last girl to leave the dormitory that first morning and only then, realised, after gazing around, that her uniform brown dress was very faded compared with the crisp, new dresses that the other girls were wearing. The dress was more mustard, than brown, having been washed on numerous occasions. Emma was feeling very ill at ease as she hurried out of the junior dormitory.

She caught up with the last of the stragglers, following them into the refectory, before diverting to her table. No-one said anything to her about her dress although some were looking her up and down. Emma wanted to shrivel into obscurity. As soon as grace was said, the little old nun who'd rung the bell in the dormitory and whose name Emma found out was Mother Teresa, beckoned Emma. She stood up and sheepishly left the table amidst the stares of the other occupants, making her way passed the other tables to where the nun was waiting. She felt that all eyes were on her and flushed crimson.

'Come with me, dear,' Mother Teresa said, gently. She led Emma upstairs. Emma didn't know why she was picked out but didn't dare ask. She meekly followed the nun, full of trepidation and anxiety. They eventually arrived at a large, wardrobe type cupboard at the end of the second corridor. Inside were dozens of shelves, each laden with neatly folded, items of uniform. 'You can't wear that dress, dear,' she voiced quietly. Mother Teresa took out a new dress and held it up against Emma. 'This one looks about right in length. Slip that one off and put this one on.' Emma silently complied. She didn't know what else she could do. 'Now, that's much better. I'll dispose of this one and you keep that one. Off you go now and get your breakfast. Think you can find your way to the refectory?' Emma nodded. She didn't dare ask who was paying for the new dress, but she knew her mam couldn't afford it. All she could do, she thought, was to explain what happened when letter writing time came, on Saturday.

With great speed, Emma made her way back down the stairs and on arriving at the refectory, pushed open the door. Many pairs of eyes looked her way. For a moment, the noise lulled as the girls noticed the change of dress, before the chatter and laughter recommenced. She wished she was invisible as she sidled to her table and sat down. There was a hard-boiled egg in front of her, almost cold. The tea was strong and sweet.
'I don't take sugar in my tea,' Emma ventured, looking up to Judith.
'I'm sorry, but you don't have a choice,' Judith responded. 'The tea comes from the large tea urn over there on that table. We take turns, table by table, week by week following a rota, to go to the urn and fill our cups. We were almost the last today and consequently the tea is rather strong. It's already sweetened.' Emma drank some and thought it was vile.
'Not like our tea at home,' she thought, 'very weak and with lots of milk in it but no sugar.' She took the last half slice of

bread and margarine to eat with her cold egg and breakfast was over. The same ritual that took place the night before, of standing in silence and saying thanksgiving grace, was repeated and likewise, of walking in single line and in silence to the chapel.

After morning prayers in the chapel, Emma followed the others up the stairs to the dormitory. In the junior dormitory, the girls were making their beds. She walked to her own bed, pulled the covers up and pushed her pyjamas under the pillow. After taking her pen, pencil, rubber and ruler from her locker, she followed one or two girls back to the boarders' room, not knowing quite what else to do. One after the other, girls sauntered in and soon there was quite a lot of noise. 'Everyone seems to know someone to talk to,' thought Emma, glancing around at huddles of girls chattering and laughing, still catching up with their holiday stories. There were a handful who seemed unsure and apprehensive like she was feeling.

Whilst standing there, she was approached by a tall, slightly built, older girl. As the girl came closer, Emma noticed her pale blue eyes and cropped, blond hair and her pleasant smile.
'Hello, you are Emma, aren't you?' she questioned. Emma nodded. 'I'm Maureen and I'm head of the boarders which means I'm around to especially help our new starters with any concerns. When I checked the junior dormitory just now, I noticed that your bed isn't made properly.'
'Well, I just did it like I do at home,' Emma responded, nervously. She was feeling weepy.
'It's okay. I'll take you and show you how to do it correctly,' replied Maureen, sympathetically. 'Come on. Follow me. Just leave your pens on the table. We won't be long.'

So, for the second time, Emma left the others and this time went with the senior girl up the stairs to the dormitory feeling that she wanted to explain a bit more.
'You see,' she said, as they approached the dormitory, 'we don't have anywhere much to put stuff away at home and our bed, that I share with Martha, is always messy with clothes and we just tidy it a bit before getting into bed.' At

this, her lip started trembling, on mentioning her sister's name. They entered the junior dormitory. Glancing around the room, Emma noticed that all the other beds were neatly made compared to hers.

'Every morning, after breakfast, you come back to the dormitory and make your bed like this,' Maureen explained, as she remade the bed. 'Have you a pyjama case?' Emma shook her head. 'Well, fold the pyjamas very neatly and carefully place them under your pillow. On Mass mornings, we make our beds after Mass but before breakfast. Okay?' Emma nodded.

'Thank you for coming with me,' she whispered.

'Don't worry. It's fine. Now you need to go to the main hall where we were at recreation last night and join the other pupils. Pick up your pens from the boarders' room, on your way.' Emma rushed off, hoping she would be able to find the hall. She went to the boarders' room first, for her pen, pencil, rubber and ruler and was pleased to see the last of the girls coming out. She caught them up and kept close to them wondering if she would ever get used to the maze of corridors and flights of stairs.

Arriving in the large school hall, Emma met with a din of voices and a sea of faces. She was aghast. There were hundreds of girls of all shapes and sizes. The pupils were chattering like magpies on their first day back. Emma was used to her village school with thirty or so children of all ages in one classroom with the same teacher as only rarely was the second classroom used with the help of another teacher. 'This is a nightmare,' she thought.

She gingerly pushed her way through the milling girls, trying to find a familiar face from the night before. She said a mental prayer, her only hope of consolation in her predicament, as she searched this way and that. At last, she saw Faith and smiled. 'Thank God,' she thought. Faith smiled back. 'I am pleased to see you,' Emma ventured, her lip trembling, feeling so relieved that she was almost on the verge of tears. She pulled herself together and stood close by Faith. She noticed that Faith's wavy, auburn hair was now very neatly plaited and hanging well down her back. She had lots of freckles too, which Emma thought very attractive.

'Who does your hair like that? It's lovely and thick, isn't it,' she commented. Faith smiled.
'Thank you. The little nun who rings the bell in the dormitory plaited it for me this morning. She's ever so sweet and gentle.'

A bell rang loudly. The noise subsided. Mother Monica, straight as a ramrod, walked onto the stage followed by a procession of a few nuns and several ladies whom Emma decided must be the teachers. She noticed that some of the ladies were wearing a long, black, kind of cloak over their dress or suit.
'I must ask about those,' she thought, wondering what they were.
'We will begin with prayers and then I will call out a teacher's name followed by names of pupils. When you hear your name called, step forward and when told, follow your teacher to your form room in a silent orderly fashion, please. Remember to assemble here each morning, each form in its own line for prayers. You are not allowed to go to your form rooms before assembly.' Emma listened carefully. She heard her name announced and joined a long row of young girls who were headed by a tubby, little nun with glasses. The nun was wearing a black full-length dress with the added narrow blue piece of cloth hanging down, like Mother Monica. She noticed Audrey in the line but no other boarder. Then Faith's name was called out and she walked over to join the line, smiling at Emma who'd turned her head to see her. Emma was so pleased that Faith was in her form. At least she would know two others.

The nun in charge of their form must have had her list of the girls with her because when Mother Monica paused for a moment, she turned and walked through the door at the far end of the hall and down a corridor. The girls followed. On arriving at their form room, the pupils scrambled to sit in pairs at the double desks. Emma looked around for Faith, but she was speaking with Audrey and they were already seated side by side. She knew they lived in the same town and they'd obviously chosen to sit together. Emma saw that the places were filling up. She spotted an empty seat next to a rather overweight girl.

'Can I sit next to you please?' The girl smiled and nodded and introduced herself.

'I'm Peg.'

'Thank you. I'm Emma, one of the new boarders,' Emma responded, grateful that she was finally seated.

Emma noticed, when looking around, that some of the girls wore plain brown V-neck identical cardigans whereas her cardigan was a deep brown, cable-patterned, high neck button-up. She was so proud of it when Mary, having spent hour after hour in the evenings by the light of the Tilley lamp in the farmhouse kitchen knitting it for her, finally finished it. She'd explained, at the time, that the uniform was so expensive at the special shop in Scarborough where it was available, that it was cheaper to knit one. Emma thought the cardigan was beautiful. She'd decided not to wear it yet as it was a warm September day and she'd left it in her bedside locker. She was so glad she'd done that as she realised it would have been embarrassing for her had she worn it, as it was so different from the standard uniform cardigan. 'Maybe I'll manage without it until half-term and mam might give me money to go to the shop for a proper uniform one,' she thought, hopefully. 'I will be able to wear my brown knitted one in the evenings if it comes in cooler. So, it will still be good to have it,' she decided, thinking this would please her mam.

There was a tapping sound. The nun, sitting at the front facing them, was trying to get their attention by rapping on her desk.

'Good morning. Settle down, please. Are you all seated?' One or two latecomers were sidling in and taking whatever seats were available. 'I'm Mother Catherine, your form teacher. This is Form II. I have a list here of your names in alphabetical order. I need from each of you your father's name and your address please. This information is for your report books.' She held one up to demonstrate her point, showing the girls the first page where such details were to be written. 'When I have completed the form, come and take your report book, pick up a sheet of brown paper from my desk and return to your place and back it and write your name on the front. They will all be collected at the end of this session. These report books are distributed on the last day of term, each subject giving your term and exam marks and your overall position. The teachers of each subject add their remarks on your efforts for the term, plus there will be a comment on your general attendance and conduct. Mother Monica, the head teacher, reads and signs each report. You take them home to be signed by a parent or guardian and then bring them back to school to your form room at the beginning of the following term.' Emma listened carefully.

Mother Catherine began with the first name on her list. Emma was fascinated by the different addresses, but none were like hers.

'58 Peasholm Way, Scarborough,' said Peg, on hearing her name called out.

'29 Quayside, Scarborough,' said another.

'91 Marine Avenue, Scarborough.'

'7 St John Street.' There were many more. Then it was her turn.

'Emma Holmes. Your father's name please.'

'Tom.'

'Is his full name Thomas?' Mother Catherine questioned.

'Yes, but he gets Tom.' The nun wrote it down. Some of the girls turned to look at Emma.

'And your address, please.'

'Bankside farm,' Emma started, and the nun interjected.

'Is Bankside one word?'

'Yes.'

'Yes, Mother,' the nun instructed. 'And the next line?'

'Moorbeck.'

'One word or two?'

'One,' replied Emma, beginning to feel embarrassed as more and more heads were turning her way. Eyes were staring at her.

'Then what?' Mother Catherine was sounding a little impatient.

'Windrush. It's just one word,' ventured Emma, blushing a deep red and wishing she could hide away somewhere. Mother Catherine raised her black and grey bushy eyebrows.

'And the town?' questioned the nun, 'and that will do.'

'Whitby,' and with that, Emma hung her head and gazed

down at her desk. 'I was going to say that next, if she'd just waited,' she thought. 'Why do I have to be so different?'

At last, the reports were completed and collected. Mother Catherine called forward a girl to hand out to each pupil a timetable of their weekly lessons specifying in which room they were held when not in their own form room. Emma learnt that there were other rooms for some lessons such as Music and Biology. It was a long day for her with a different teacher for each subject and with exercise books piling up. The first task each pupil carried out at the beginning of every lesson was to back an exercise book and write on it their name and the subject. As the day went on, she noticed that most of the girls possessed satchels in which to put their books and pens. Emma placed hers by the side of her desk as she didn't have a satchel.

At the end of the day, she carried hers in her hands. She guessed a satchel wasn't on the list of essentials and the money from the council that paid her fees did not cover non-essentials. Tom and Mary probably didn't think about one. She was trying to remember what kind of bag Tim carried his books in when he left the farmhouse each morning to walk over the moor track to the tarmac road to catch a bus into Whitby. Emma also realised that when they'd had a geography lesson and were instructed to draw a map of Great Britain that having colouring pencils helped as some of the girls coloured in theirs in, but she didn't have any. 'Maybe someone will lend me one or two when I need to use them,' she thought. She sighed. She was glad when classes were finally over. She couldn't see any way of getting colouring pencils until half-term. It seemed a lifetime away and Emma was beginning to wonder if she would survive that long. She was longing for Moorbeck and to be with her family. She was fighting tears again.

Emma carried her books along the corridors and up flights of stairs to the boarders' room and put them in her locker. There were other girls milling about and she followed them down to the vestry, too tired to make conversation. It was time for the obligatory daily walk. She remembered Joanne telling her about this daily excursion. She made her way around some boarders in the throes of changing into their outdoor shoes and brushed past others struggling to put on their coats, eventually finding her peg. After putting on her coat and hat and feeling glad that no-one seemed to notice the patch on her coat pocket, she changed her shoes, making sure she placed her indoor ones in the wooden cubby-hole. She then mingled among the girls walking down the corridor to a side entrance of the convent which led directly onto the street. Here, they congregated and mostly paired up whilst awaiting a nun to shepherd them on this, their first of many daily walks.

'I could do with some fresh air,' thought Emma. 'It might help to keep me going.' Joanne noticed Emma looking a little lost and went to speak with her.
'How are you doing?' she whispered. 'Have you managed today?' Emma nodded. She didn't want to say how she was really feeling in front of the others. 'Unfortunately, you won't see much of me during the day except possibly at break time as our form room is on a different corridor to yours,' Joanne explained. She was remembering that she'd told her mother she would help Emma settle in, but their paths didn't cross much during school hours. Even at break times, Joanne was with her own peer group. 'At weekends,' Joanne continued, 'the walk is a much longer one and is at a different time. We go on more interesting ones and we don't have to stay in line so much. You'll enjoy those. You'll soon get into the routine,' she added, reassuringly.

Another nun arrived. One that Emma had not seen before. Later, she learnt that this nun taught at the preparatory school at Normanton Rise, in a different location of Scarborough, where younger children attended before coming to the convent school.
'Maybe that's where Susanna went,' she thought, remembering what Mother Monica said about Susanna being a boarder last year. 'She would have been too young to be at the grammar school. It must have been hard for her coming to a boarding school at such a young age,' she pondered, feeling some sympathy for Susanna. A voice interrupted her thoughts.
'Come along,' Emma heard the nun say and realised it was

to her that the nun was referring. She stepped out of the side door and onto the street.

'Not like stepping out of our door at home. We just step onto the cobbles but see nothing but green fields and cows and a farm or two away in the distance.' She gulped. 'Don't cry,' she told herself. 'It's just because you're tired.'

With older ones leading the way, a crocodile of girls, dressed in brown, began walking down Queen Street, with the nun bringing up the rear. It was a common sight each day in the town to see a procession of boarders walking the streets or in the parks or along the beaches. At the beginning of this term, the older girls with friends, easily paired off, as did one or two new ones who were beginning to recognise others and were walking side by side. Anyone without a partner stayed back with the nun or walked in front of her with another partner-less girl. On this first occasion, Emma hadn't anyone as Faith, whom she would like to have partnered, was chatting to her companion, Audrey. She hung back to walk with another loner, in front of the nun with her long black dress and its blue over-piece.

'It must be the teachers who have that extra piece of blue cloth hanging down,' Emma was thinking, having mulled this over, 'as those nuns we see who work in the kitchen in the basement don't have them.' She found it an effort to make conversation with someone she didn't know but the alternative was a silence that was embarrassing. She tried but struggled throughout the walk and was glad to be back at the convent.

Inside again to change back into indoor shoes and after taking off her hat and coat, Emma followed the others to the dormitories. She took off her uniform, folded it carefully ready for tomorrow and put on her own clothes before heading, in silence, to the refectory for tea. She wanted to leap down the broad, shallow stairs, three at a time for the sheer joy of it but remembered to walk each step as instructed. There was a little hushed whispering after grace as the girls were settling down at the tables.

'I hope you've all had a good first day and are not too tired,' said Judith, at the head of the table.

'Have any of you brought any extras?' she asked them, glancing from girl to girl. Emma's face was a blank. Something else that she was unaware of. The responses flowed in.

'I've brought a swiss roll.'

'I've a jar of marmite in my locker upstairs. I'll bring it down next time.'

'My mother gave me a pot of home-made jam.'

'Dad bought some apples for me, but I left them in the boarders' room.'

Emma remained silent.

'We all bring extra food to be shared,' explained Judith, noticing the anxious look on her face. 'Today, we're having the cake that I brought. We get either jam or cake for tea but not both and so the extras help a bit. When you come back after half-term, maybe you can bring something or if someone visits you one Saturday, perhaps you can ask for something.' Emma nodded. She didn't think anyone would be coming to visit her, which was allowed on a Saturday or Sunday. With Mother Monica's permission, boarders were even allowed out with their visitor for an hour or two, so long as they were back for tea. Mary explained this to her daughter on the bus when they were travelling to the convent, but Emma knew what an effort that would be for her parents and anyway, they always had too much to do on the farm.

'Yes, I can ask at half-term,' Emma replied to Judith, 'but I don't think anyone from home will be visiting as they're too busy and they don't have a car and it's a long way,' she added. Judith smiled her acknowledgement but didn't comment. Emma was wondering if her mam would be able to afford to buy an extra but didn't like to say that. The cake, that Judith placed on the table, was delicious. It was a very thick one with chocolate filling through it. It was shared out equally amongst the six around the table. Other than that, there was only bread and jam for tea. After grace at the end of the plain meal, the girls streamed out in silence and back upstairs to the boarders' room.

Emma took her homework from her locker and found a place at the table where Faith and Audrey were sitting. Smiling at them, she opened her English exercise book and proceeded to think about how to approach the task set by the English teacher. She finished the piece of work and was wondering how to fill in the time when Mother Teresa, who was supervising and whom Emma remembered from the night before, called out to say that pupils from Year II and under could go to recreation for half an hour. It was then that Emma realised that Susanna must be in Year I as she was a year younger than Emma.

'No rushing and please be quiet as there are others trying to work,' the nun reminded them. Girls at various tables stood up, moved their chairs in and made for the door, including Faith and Audrey. Emma followed them. A nun led them into another room and the girls sat around, some chatting whilst others, having remembered to take a book, were soon quietly engrossed reading. Emma found it hard going and boring. Susanna was the only bright spark and entertained anyone who cared to listen with stories of her previous escapades at the prep school, as she called it. Emma thought she must have been quite troublesome for the teachers.

They returned to the boarders' room to join the older girls until supper time at twenty minutes past seven o'clock. Emma, having finished the little homework she'd been given, doodled in her jotting book to pass the time. She thought it was good to have a jotter to doodle in, even though this was not exactly the reason they'd been given them. Each pupil was issued with one for rough work when problems arose around homework such as maths calculations. The nun rang the bell much to her relief and the girls cleared away their books and lined up to go downstairs for supper. Again, the silent walk to the refectory and then afterwards to chapel for night prayers finishing with the hymn *Lead Kindly Light*. As the words of the third verse, *the night is dark and I am far from home*, were sung, Emma could take no more. She finally gave way to the tears that she'd been suppressing all day. The words continued, *o'er moor and fen, o'er crag and torrent till...*' and Emma couldn't see, as her eyes were filling up and the lights started winking and blinking as she tried to focus. She struggled and swallowed and regained control, but it was short-lived. Eventually, as the hymn ended,

Emma, wiping her eyes and blowing her nose, fought back further tears and regained her composure as the girls streamed out of chapel.

It was later, when Emma finally disappeared under the bed clothes in her pyjamas, that she really let go and silently sobbed and sobbed as if her heart would break. She longed to fling her arms around her dad and have a kiss from Mary and play with her brothers and sisters, especially Martha. She yearned for a run over the pastures or a walk on the moor. The ache in her heart was so strong and her pillow was becoming quite wet with the hot, salty tears that would not cease. She finally fell asleep, her body still twitching and jumping from the silent sobs.

****

'That was weeks ago,' thought Emma, as she found herself still clutching Martha's letter in her hand, 'and I've learnt so much since then.' The memories of wakening early that second morning, lying in bed and thinking about her predicament, were still very vivid, with her eyes feeling puffy from the tears she'd shed. She remembered thinking that she just had to keep going, focusing on her dad, Tom, and deciding to try and be like him. It was Tom's resilient nature that pulled him through many rough months following his arrival, with Mary, a town girl, and their three little ones, at Bankside farm with little money or stock or farm machinery. Three more children were born in the draughty farmhouse and conditions were tough. Those early years were of poverty and hardship and Emma, the third of the children, was brought up alongside her siblings with this determination to succeed under whatever situations arose because that's what Tom always said. She had neither the money nor many clothes nor was she as well-equipped, such as having colouring pencils and a satchel, as many of her peer group at this school, but she decided that she wouldn't give in but try and make the best of it.

So that morning, after the attack of homesickness the previous evening, Emma quietly washed, dressed and went down to breakfast with the others. No-one commented when she arrived at table with very puffy eyes. She's doused them with cold water at the wash basin, but they were still swollen and rather red. She chose to ignore any stares and occupied herself, eating whilst others chatted.

As each day passed, it became easier settling into the routine. Emma's peer group found her to be cheerful and pleasant and she was popular because she was always ready to listen. She was also a hard worker and soon stood out as one of the cleverer girls, particularly at Maths. 'Emma, how do you work this out?' was the question invariably asked of her before the maths teacher arrived. In the boarders' room at night, the pupils of Emma's age were often asking permission from the supervising nun, to speak with her as they wanted help with their homework.
'I don't understand this algebra.'
'Can you show me how to draw this angle?'
'What does this English question mean?' Emma was pleased to help. Her confidence in herself was growing.

The day girls in her Form were interested in Emma because she seemed different. Apart from Faith and Audrey, they were all town girls living in or near to Scarborough. Even Faith and Audrey lived in a town, albeit a smaller market town but still with a swimming pool and picture house and many shops. Although the day girls teased Emma sometimes, they were also fascinated by her description of her home life and were intrigued by some of her responses to their questions over these early weeks.
'Haven't you really got a television?' one asked in surprise.
'We've no electricity. So, we can't have one.'
'Well, what do you do for lights?' another questioned.
'We take candles to bed. Downstairs we have a Tilley lamp that hangs from a beam in the kitchen.' There was a lull as the girls tried to take this in before returning to their seats as the teacher walked in.

'And you've never been to the swimming baths?' queried another, in amazement, on another occasion. Faith was listening in as the day pupils questioned Emma whilst they were waiting for the geography teacher to arrive for first lesson of the day. She shook her head. Faith was astounded at some of her replies.

'Don't you ever go to the pictures?' she asked Emma, remembering the many visits to the pictures with her mam. Faith couldn't imagine what life would be like without visits to a picture house. Emma admitted to not going. She didn't know what film stars were. The day girls were staggered. Most of them went to the cinema regularly.

'What do you do at night and at weekends?' Peg questioned, early one afternoon. Although normally a very quiet girl, Peg felt confident about asking as she still shared a desk with Emma. She'd listened carefully to the conversations and was curious about life without any of the out of school activities that the others mentioned. Emma gave this question some thought, looking at her attentive audience at the time and wondering quite how to explain. She decided to go for it and told her listeners something of what farm life is like and how the children helped with weeding turnips, milking cows, gathering eggs and cleaning out calf-pens and at hay time.

'Every night in winter, my dad has to do up and I help if I'm not minding our little ones for my mam.' The girls were looking puzzled as they hadn't understood some of what she said. 'You mention about your dad doing up. Doing up what? What does that mean?' Peg questioned. She was genuinely interested as she thought Emma's life sounded a lot more exciting than her own.

They waited whilst Emma struggled to put her thoughts into words.
Well,' she began, very tentatively, wondering quite how to explain, 'in winter, cows stay inside the cowshed and of course they poo and wee and their bedding becomes wet and dirty. It has to be shovelled out and fresh bedding put down.'
'Bedding. What's that?' queried someone.
'It just means the straw that the cows lie on.'
'And you have to shift it all when they've messed on it?' chirped up another girl.
'Yes, it's what you do on a farm.'
'That's disgusting,' someone commented.
'Well, don't any of you lot help with washing pots and cleaning shoes and tidying up?' Emma questioned, looking

over at Audrey who was listening intently. Audrey shook her head. She was an only child and didn't do any of that. She was still pondering over other things that Emma told them. 'You mentioned about planting seeds but grass just grows, doesn't it,' she stated, adamantly. There were a few nods in the circle.

'No, it doesn't, not hay anyway,' retorted Emma. 'The soil has to be prepared, manured, spread with fertilizer and seeds planted.' As usual, the conversation ceased on the arrival of the teacher.

'I'll have to tell them later about playing cards at night and having sing-songs,' thought Emma, opening her exercise book. Otherwise it sounds like all work, but we do have fun.

Faith didn't understand Emma's earlier comments the previous day, about cows drying up. She knew that milk came from cows. She thought everyone knew that, but she had a query.

'What did you mean when you said that a cow dries up?' she questioned, later in the day, whilst the girls were hanging around in the form room waiting for the English teacher to arrive. Some of them edged forward to listen.

'Well, when a cow has a calf, it gives pints and pints of milk, morning and night, sometimes even at lunch time in the early days after calving, but as the months go by, the cow produces less and less. Eventually the milk dries up, but by this time the cow's heavy in calf again. After the calf is born, the cow gives lots of milk again. And it just goes on. It's nature, of course.' Emma knew the signs when a cow was 'a-bulling' too, but she didn't expect them to know and she thought maybe this wasn't the right time to go into it.

Apart from The Farmers Weekly, her knowledge from newspapers, television and the cinema was dismal, but she more than held her own when farming life was discussed. Not that the topic was raised very often, but on the occasions when it arose, her peer group were finding her to be quite an interesting person despite her strange accent. Emma just felt an odd one out and didn't enjoy it much. Suddenly the door opened. The girls moved quickly to their desks as the teacher walked in, in a fluster as she was a little late.

'Good morning. Settle down please. Books out. We'll continue from where we left off on Friday.' There was no opportunity for more explanations and Emma was glad. She felt that she had been bombarded with questions and was happy to bury herself into the English lesson instead of explaining more about her personal family life.

It was later that same week when the girls were having a cookery lesson in the domestic science room, that Emma was acutely embarrassed at comments on her pronunciation of some words.

'What did you say?' questioned Audrey, standing nearby. 'I've put fud in't uvin, Why? What's wrong?' There were peals of laughter from other girls nearby. The teacher came across to quieten the girls and told them to get on with their work. Emma was mortified. She usually joined in when the girls were laughing at her but inwardly, it upset her a lot. By laughing, she was pretending not to care as she was determined not to show how she was really feeling. 'Why did they all laugh? What did I say?' she whispered to Faith, whilst they were at the sink together washing their cooking utensils.

'It isn't what you say but how you say it. You don't say *fud*. It's pronounced *food* and you don't say *in't uvin* but *in the oven*,' replied Faith, laughing quietly at her own attempt at the broad Yorkshire accent.

Faith was taking elocution lessons and explained to Emma that the tutor was teaching her how to pronounce words correctly, even though she didn't have a noticeable accent. Emma was silent. She thought that she would need to listen more as to how some words were pronounced and be extra careful when she was speaking. She remembered Mary saying something to Tom about the nun advising elocution lessons but, at the time, didn't understand what the nun meant. Now she realised that elocution meant speaking correctly. Maybe she'd ask in her letter home if she could have some of those lessons. She didn't like being laughed at. If she explained to her mam, maybe they'd find the money as elocution lessons were extras to be paid for.

Other extras were horse riding, ballet or music lessons which some of the boarders took. She remembered seeing a list of names on the notice board in the boarders' room of those who took music lessons. Alongside each name was the allocated room in which they went to practise in the evening and once, when she went to the toilet from the boarders' room, she saw one of the older boarders playing at a piano as the girl had left the door slightly ajar. Emma couldn't imagine doing ballet. She'd seen ballerinas in a book that Audrey lent her. She was a bit scared of horses and was not inclined to ride one. Piano lessons didn't appeal to her either although she enjoyed singing, but elocution seemed a worthwhile activity.

There were highlights in Emma's busy week, one of which was having a bath. As there were only five bathrooms for the girls, all their names were listed on the notice board in the boarders' room with a weekly allocated half-an-hour bath time aside each name. Taking a bath was a new experience for Emma, with the taps running and the water getting higher and higher. She thought it was absolute bliss lying in warm water and topping it up as the water cooled down. She relished the break from studying and looked forward to her weekly bath. Hair washing was once a fortnight as instructed by Mother Monica, but Emma noticed some of the older girls with wet hair every time they went for a bath. She didn't dare break the rule though. Bath time for her was every Wednesday evening whereupon she left the boarders' room with four other girls after asking permission to leave from the supervising nun and stating their reason. She discovered that three of the older girls in the group had their favourite bathroom, but she didn't mind at all which one she used. A bath was a bath and she lazed in it for as long as was allowed, soaking up the warmth and enjoying the comfort it brought her, alone with her thoughts. She was happy.

Saturdays were a pleasure too for Emma because it was when she received a letter from home. Everyday Mother Monica came into the refectory carrying a small stack of letter and sometimes a parcel or two. It was post for the boarders. As each name was read out and Mother handed a letter over, every pair of eyes was looking with hopeful expectation on the pile of letters becoming smaller and smaller.

'Will there be one for me,' was each girl's thought. Some girls received parcels and others, letters twice a week, but Emma knew she wouldn't get a letter during the week. She waited in anticipation, every Saturday morning, for her name to be called out, as that was the day her mam's letter arrived. Mary always wrote in a rush on a Friday morning, apologising for the shortness of the letter but that she needed to finish it before the postman arrived. Living on an isolated farm on the Yorkshire moors meant that the mail didn't arrive until later in the day, but at least she didn't need to make a journey to post her letter as the postmen were very obliging and happy to take letters to the sorting office on their return to the depot. Mary struggled to find time to write to her daughter, with helping on the farm and looking after her many children, but she felt it important that Emma received a weekly letter and hence her rush on Fridays to make sure that it was ready for when the postman arrived.

I'm sorry for the shortness again, her mam wrote in this latest letter, *but you know how it is, seeing the children off to school, taking your dad his morning mug of tea to the cowshed as well as getting Jacob dressed to take with me as he's too little to stay in the house on his own. Sometimes I'm helping your dad, when he wants a hand. I don't seem to get around to writing until later in the day. I'll try and write more next time…* Emma knew it was an effort for her mam and that she meant to write more. She continued reading. *We love getting your letter each week. You seem to have a busy life. Won't it be lovely at half-term when you can come home for a few days. Martha is missing you a lot…* Even though the letters were short, they were still letters and Emma was happy just to receive one. She wondered though if her mam realised just how important that weekly letter was – not to be forgotten, to know that back on Bankside farm, she was still thought about. On some occasions, the letter arrived on the Friday after Mary made an effort to write earlier in the week and this surprise brought great delight to Emma. She never read hers at table like some of the girls but preferred to read them in private.

The letter writing was a two-way occurrence because every Saturday the boarders were instructed to write to their parents and there was an allotted time for this. After writing the letters, the girls left them on the table, occupied by the nun-in-charge, to be posted later. The new boarders were told not to stick down the envelope as Mother Monica read them before they were sealed. Emma hated the thought of her letter being read by a nun and was careful what she put in it. She didn't mention about her homesickness as she didn't want the nun to know and anyway, she knew it would be upsetting for her parents, but she wrote about her lessons and the walks.

After some weeks passed, these girls were told that they could seal their own letters. Emma supposed that the nun wanted to make sure nothing critical was being written about the school or the conditions under which they lived. As well as leaving her written letter open, she noticed that the letter received from her mam was also not sealed. She felt uncomfortable about this too, but within a few weeks, the letter handed to her was still sealed, no doubt because Mother Monica recognised Mary's writing.

It was during the exchange of letters that Mary informed Emma of the elocution lessons planned for her, this a result of Emma explaining to Mary about the need to improve her pronunciation of words. She was delighted to join Faith in taking advantage of these extra lessons and they went together to see the tutor one session a week after dinner but before afternoon school classes began. Faith was much more confident than she was and seemed to enjoy the opportunity to stand up and recite verses to the tutor. On the other hand, Emma found it quite uncomfortable being corrected on the many words that she was speaking incorrectly. She hated standing there, feeling embarrassed and ill at ease.
'I daren't miss them,' she thought, 'as I know they are expensive. I'll stick it out till Christmas and then tell mam that I don't want to go any more. She'll understand.'
'It will get easier,' Faith reassured her on their way back to their form room, one Tuesday afternoon, 'and you won't get teased as much by the other girls then,' she added,

comfortingly. 'I found it hard at first, but I've been going since the start of term and you can see how confident I am now.'

The word *teased* reminded Emma of the previous day when waiting for the nun to join them for the daily walk. It was when one of a small group of giggling girls, decided to pick on her.

'She's got a real monkey face, hasn't she,' the girl laughingly said, loud enough for Emma to hear, 'with her shiny, black, short-cut hair and those heavy, beetling, black eyebrows.'
'I was thinking more of a rabbit. Haven't you noticed her buck teeth?' added another voice. Emma grinned because she didn't know what else to do. She felt very small and alone as no-one else seem to hear or else they chose to ignore it. She wanted to curl up inside herself.
'Going shopping, are you,' quipped another, 'with those bags under your eyes when you smile?' After getting no response, the three girls in question turned their attention to another youngster before the nun finally arrived and everyone streamed out onto the street.

'That's a relief,' thought Emma, making sure she was well away from the tormentors as she didn't know how to deal with their comments.
Apart from letter-writing, there were other regular chores on Saturdays that were part of the routine for the boarders, one of which was shoe cleaning. Both shoe cleaning and sewing equipment were among the list of essentials that each boarder was required to have. The wooden stairs to the attic were taken up each Saturday morning by boarders sitting on them, cleaning and polishing their shoes but this was one time when chatting was permitted. Emma was well practised in shoe cleaning as one of her jobs on the farm on Saturdays was to clean all the shoes.

At home, having scraped all the dirt off the shoes onto pages torn out of an old Farmers Weekly, she brushed on the polish and gave the shoes a good shine. When she'd finished cleaning and polishing them, she placed them, a pair at a time, on each of the stair steps so that Tom and Mary and her siblings could easily find them when getting ready for church on Sundays. It was a tedious job at home because there was plenty of muck around that was picked up when wearing the shoes, but Emma was quite proud of how shiny the shoes were, when she finished. Having two pairs to clean at the convent was an easy chore for her and she found herself helping some of the other new boarders who had never tackled such a job before.

Later, on a Saturday morning, was mending time in the boarders' room. Every fortnight, each boarder placed their dirty washing inside a pillowcase and put it outside their cubicle curtain, or on their bed in sight, to make sure it was collected. The clean laundry was inspected by a nun before being returned and any items in need of repair were removed. As each item was labelled, the removed items of clothing were handed out to their owners on the alternate Saturdays to be mended. The rule of silence was lifted at weekends and for those who had not been given any sewing, it was free time to chat or read.

As well as being adept at shoe cleaning, Emma was also a neat sewer, again having had plenty of practise at home especially at darning socks.
'Will you darn this for me please. I'll give you a few sweets on Sunday,' was often asked of her by Audrey, being an only child and not practised in these tedious chores. Polly was another who asked for help with sewing. She had one younger brother, Emma learnt, and came from further South. She frequently received parcels as did Audrey and they seemed to be chumming up together.
'They're pleasant enough,' Emma thought, 'but different from me. However, she didn't mind helping them especially if given sweets.

On one Saturday, Margaret, the bonny girl with freckles whom Emma met on the stairs on her first day, came over to her.
'Will you darn one of my socks, please? How did you learn to do it so neatly?'
'My mam taught me. I darn a lot at home. Great big holes that sometimes slipped over the edge of the wooden mushroom that I hold in the sock. I use a mushroom so that I don't catch the rest of the sock with the needle.'

'Well, I can darn, but not like you. You must have practised a lot.'

'I have five brothers and sisters and my mam can't afford new things and we just mend or patch clothes and stitch or darn our socks.' Margaret was smiling at her.

'Thank you. You've done that so well whilst we've been chatting.'

'Good, isn't she,' said Mother Teresa who was over-seeing the girls and was listening to this conversation. Emma felt a little glow inside herself.

After the busy Saturday morning, the boarders went for lunch and then congregated at the side door in anticipation of a long walk around Scarborough, a resort with plenty of interesting places to be explored, not only by the locals, but by the many holiday makers too. As well as sporting two coves with lengthy stretches of sand, the town offered a stroll along the Marine Drive, or a saunter through some beautiful parks, Peasholm Park being a particularly enjoyable one. Other interesting explorations were the zig-zag paths down to the sands or the playground near the old castle with a wooded area around it.

Emma looked forward to the Saturday walk, a highlight in her life at present, because although the boarders set off as usual in their crocodile line, they were permitted to break out of the line when once arriving at their chosen destination of the day. She particularly liked the castle walk, which they'd done once before, climbing the grassy banks or playing hide and seek with some of the younger boarders, in and out of the bushes and through the undergrowth surrounding the castle, or having a turn on the swings and roundabouts in a play area nestled alongside the wooded area.

On other occasions, she loved the sense of freedom when running along the sands and was one of the braver ones who walked on the large sewer pipes that lead out to sea, visible when the tide was out, but this was done discreetly as Mother didn't approve. On that specific walk, Emma enjoyed the fresh, salty sea air all around her whilst watching the sea pound along the shore. She thought it wonderful to soak up the magnificent views across the ocean with the ships on the horizon. There was a great expanse of rocks to be investigated and walked on and she loved stepping across the rocks covered in seaweed and little pebbles, thus avoiding the little pools of water in between.

These visits reminded Emma of home and their annual trip to the sands with her mam and her brothers and sisters. It was always such an adventure, the one day in the summer holidays when they walked the mile over the moor to catch a bus to the nearest beach, carrying their egg sandwiches and their diluted, welfare orange juice drinks. The excursion was a real treat. Waves of homesickness flooded her when she thought of those happy times but, pushing them aside, she continued enjoying the release from the rigid discipline and silences and hard days at school, as did many of the girls, especially the younger ones. They laughed and talked and ran around until they were ushered back to the nun by older girls.

Sunday was another very different day from the weekdays. Although like Saturdays regarding discipline being relaxed over the crocodile line once away from the main streets of Scarborough, it was the afternoon that was very special. After dinner, the girls all returned to the boarders' room and broke up into groups chatting, some going to their lockers to get out puzzle or reading books. Others brought out sketch books. Audrey even had a board game and gathered a few around her to play and sometimes Emma joined in.

This activity continued until Mother Monica, or whoever was her replacement to supervise the girls, eventually walked in carrying the box of purses normally kept locked in Mother Monica's office outside the boarders' room. The nun placed the box at the far end table. She then unlocked the cupboard that stood in the corner of the boarders' room and taking from it many boxes of sweets and chocolate, spread them out over the length of the table leaving a space at one end for the box of purses. The nun also took from the cupboard a stack of ration books, placing them alongside the box of purses. Sweets were one of the commodities still rationed even though it was a few years since the second world war ended. The boarders weren't allowed to eat sweets during the week and were strictly forbidden to accept sweets from day pupils. Emma, like many others, found it difficult to refuse an offer of a sweet and these rules were discreetly broken many times.

The girls queued up in a disorderly manner, each girl claiming her own purse and her ration book and moving along the table edge, chose and paid for her favourite items, eagerly anticipating the pleasure of eating sweets again. Coupons were carefully torn out of the ration book. The nun overseeing this operation, made sure the younger girls only used their allotted coupons for the week but some of the unsupervised older girls were passing their unwanted coupons to those who indulged more. The nun was occupied selling the sweets and paid little attention to the coupons being laid in an untidy heap on the corner of the table. After each girl made her purchase, she placed her ration book on the mounting pile ready to be locked away when selling was completed and likewise, putting her purse back in the box.

Emma didn't purchase as many as some of the boarders because she needed to make her small amount of pocket money last until half-term and was aware that she must keep enough to pay for her bus fare home. She began sampling her small hoard of sweets.
'I've never seen one of these before,' she confided in Faith, holding up a stick she'd bitten at. 'It is absolutely delicious.' The item was a long, finger-thin round stick of chocolate, mixed with hard crispy ingredients and so tasty, Emma thought.
'They're called choc-sticks,' explained Faith. 'Why didn't you get more of them if you like them that much?' she queried, noticing that there was only one more in Emma's little pile of sweets.
'Well, they'd nearly all gone by the time I reached the front of the queue and I didn't like to take them all.'
'You can swop and have a couple of mine, if you like,' Faith suggested, kindly. Following this conversation, a little bartering was accomplished and both girls were happy.
Emma was beginning to feel a friendship developing towards Faith whom she found to be so gentle and with an infectious laugh.

For almost two hours, the boarders chewed and sucked their sweets with barely a break. Such was their delight at this indulgence. Towards the end of the afternoon, the supervising nun locked away the ration books and any unsold sweets ready for the following Sunday and returned the wooden box full of purses to Mother Monica's office. On re-entering the room, she immediately rang the hand bell and the girls queued to go downstairs to the refectory for tea.

'I don't feel like eating anything,' thought Emma, after consuming sweets for two hours. Although she'd finished hers earlier in the afternoon, some of the girls with plenty, had shared their sweets with her. In the refectory, the girls chatted as they nibbled at their bread sandwich but very little was eaten by anyone. They were all feeling rather sick having overindulged on so many sweets.

****

Emma dragged her thoughts back from her reminiscing, reminding herself that she needed to get out of bed.

'So much has happened over a few weeks. Martha and I will have loads of catching up to do.' She glanced over at the wash basins, but they were all occupied. 'They're taking their time again,' she thought, sighing. 'That Susanna is so slow. I hope Polly has been before her or I'll be late. I might as well finish reading this letter whilst I'm waiting,' she decided, furtively opening the pages and scanning down to the last paragraph.

You remember Mr Netherfield, don't you? Did mam tell you the latest? I guess not as they don't talk about him in front of us, but something happened not long after you went away to school. He ended up in hospital and he lent dad his van. Then he went to stay at grandad's farm to get properly better. I don't know why he went there but now he's back on his farm and dad has given him his van back and we just use the tractor again to get to church. It's still better than walking two miles, though. Dad says Jack Netherfield wasn't well when he used to drink a lot but that he's okay now and we can call him Uncle Jack instead of Mr Netherfield as he's a friend. I went with dad when he took the van back and Mr Netherfield gave me some sweets for us lot. It'll take me a while to get used to calling him Uncle Jack although he is like an uncle because he is kind to us. I'll stop now as I've run out of paper and I'm getting tired and I need to check that Jacob's all right. Martha's name was scrawled at the end and she'd added a line of kisses.

Emma thought about Mr Netherfield. She remembered that he was a bit different and unusual. He lived alone on their neighbouring farm and used to walk across the fields to call on the Holmes family occasionally. Sometimes he'd taken Mary shopping in his van which was quite a drive for him out onto a tarmac road and then joining a main road before swinging back onto the track into Moorbeck. Their mam said he was a friend, but she didn't think that her dad liked him because Tom got very cross one day and said they couldn't go to his farm anymore, but maybe that was because he'd been drinking, as dad said. She recalled him smelling of drink sometimes when she'd gone on an errand for her dad. She was pleased to read that Martha says it seems okay now between Mr Netherfield and their dad, although she wondered about the *Uncle* Jack bit.

'Maybe he is some long lost relative. He is tall and lean like dad but not as dark. Something for her and Martha to discuss,' she mused.

The news from Martha about dances, interested Emma. She thought that learning to dance would be great and wondered if any of the older boarders could dance. She'd heard of the quickstep and waltz. Maybe they could teach her at recreation time as sometimes they put records on an old gramophone when they all went to the hall after night prayers. Her thoughts were interrupted by Susanna.

'I'm finished,' she called as she was making her way to her bed, leaving Emma to give herself a very speedy wash. Emma quickly folded the letter before putting it back into the envelope and into her locker drawer.

'Only two weeks now,' she thought. 'Then I'll be back home again. Will baby Jacob remember me? Will anything be different, I wonder?'

Late Autumn 1951

The next week crept by and half-term was imminent. Emma crossed each day off in her jotter. Excitement among the boarders increased when Monday of the last week before half-term, arrived.
'Only four more nights,' she said to Faith at break time. 'Are you looking forward to going home?' Faith considered this question.
'It's quiet at our house as I only have one sister and she's quite a bit older than me. She's called Rose after my mam as she is Rose too. My three uncles live with us and are good fun, taking me fishing and hunting sometimes, but they're out a lot. They're my mam's younger brothers and are still single. So, they all share our house.'
'What about your dad, then? You never did tell me about your family last time we chatted because the bell went, if you remember.'

Faith hesitated again. Emma sensed her reluctance to speak.
'It's all right if you don't want to tell me.'
'Well, I've told you now about my uncles and my sister, Rose. Her dad died in a road accident before I was even born,' Faith answered, rather sharply, before stopping again and sighing. 'I don't like talking about this, but I don't have a dad. I suppose I have somewhere, but I've never met him. My mam changes the subject if I ask her about him. I've stopped asking her. Please don't tell anyone. My mam works in a low-paid job to bring money in and I'm on my own quite a lot. I go to the pictures to pass the time. I bet you're longing to see your brothers and sisters,' she added, changing the subject. Faith thought it sounded great having lots of siblings and envied Emma with her life on the farm and going to church on a tractor. Emma smiled and nodded but said nothing as she didn't know how to reply about Faith's home life. She couldn't imagine a life without her brothers and sisters and not having mam and dad around all the time. They walked back to their form room in silence, each lost in thoughts of such different family lives.

On Thursday evening, the air was electric as the boarders

were awaiting the arrival of Mother Monica to tell them that they could go and collect their cases from the attic and pack for their holiday break. Emma finished what little homework she'd been given. She was doodling on her jotter whilst watching the clock.

'Will Mother Monica ever come,' she wondered. The door opened and there the nun stood.

'Fifteen minutes to pack and then place your cases under the stairs near the refectory and line up for supper. Quiet please and no need to push.' This remark was a response to many of the girls jumping up and rushing to the door. Most of them could hardly restrain themselves. There were one or two who didn't go home for half-term, but Emma didn't know why. After seven weeks at school, most of them were longing to return home and were bubbling over with excitement, especially the new starters.

Emma's face was aglow. She was desperate to see her parents and brothers and sisters. Being one of the first arrivals into the attic, she found it a task hunting out her smaller case, of the two she'd brought, from the dozens in the pile. Finally scrabbling for it under a mound of cases, she pulled it free and made her way past the oncoming boarders to descend the wooden steps and into the dormitory. She quickly made her way to the junior dormitory where she packed in a few items needing washing, plus one or two spares, knowing she wouldn't need much over four days as boarders were only away from Friday to Tuesday. She intended wearing her old clothes, the ones she'd left at home, as soon as she arrived there.

'I wonder if dad will meet me off the bus with the tractor,' she thought. She'd found out that the boarders for the Whitby and Middlesbrough bus route were allowed out of classes early on the Friday afternoon to catch the tea-time bus. Her dad knew the time of arrival of the bus at Windrush road end stop. She'd written about this in her last letter home and she knew he would pick her up if he possibly could this first time. Emma felt she was going to explode with anticipation and excitement. She could hardly wait.

Next morning, there was a queue outside Mother Monica's office as the girls waited in turn to pick up their purses.

Emma was careful with her money and on being asked by the headmistress, said that she'd kept enough for her fare home. Each lesson of the day dragged for Emma. She was particularly restless and unable to pay much attention during the geography lesson in the afternoon. She kept watching the door as the call to go was imminent.

'Emma Holmes,' called out the teacher, 'will you please concentrate. I know it's half-term tonight, but we still have work to do.' Shortly, there was a knock on the form room door, before it opened to reveal one of the boarders that Emma knew was travelling on the same bus as herself. 'Please may Emma Holmes come,' the girl asked the teacher, very politely. Emma put away her books into her desk at great speed and saying goodbye, walked out of the form room, as if walking on air. The time was here!

Together the two girls walked down the corridor and then along the main one to the vestry. Maria was no taller than Emma with straight mouse-coloured hair worn with a fringe. She was nick-named *The Mouse* because of being small in stature. She was a year above Emma, in the same one as Margaret, the girl who'd asked Emma to darn a sock for her. Maria was the eldest of several children and lived in a poor area of a small town near Middlesbrough. Always a very pleasant, quietly spoken and gentle-natured girl, Maria too struggled financially. Consequently, she was very understanding of how Emma felt and was kind to her.

'Are we really going?' asked Emma, as they walked along. Maria nodded and smiled. There were a few girls already congregating in the main hall when Emma walked past to the far end of the corridor, where, under the stairs she collected her case. She returned to the vestry and put on her outdoor shoes, brown hat, coat and gloves. She was conscious of the patched pocket, but no-one had commented on it up to now. She didn't feel like explaining why it was patched and was glad that Mrs Raymons had made such a neat job of it. 'I suppose it's barely noticeable,' she thought.

It was a good walk to the bus station, the route taking them through many streets in Scarborough. On arriving there, the group of girls split up as some were travelling a different route and needed to join another bus queue leaving a handful for the Whitby and Middlesbrough stand. The girls, chattering excitedly, waiting impatiently alongside other travellers for the bus to pull in. When it arrived, the passengers dismounted first and finally the conductress and driver.

'Anyone for Middlesbrough, bring your cases,' the driver instructed, walking to the back of the bus followed by some other travellers plus three boarders including Maria. He took each of their cases and put them in the boot of the bus before disappearing into the office. Having disposed of their cases, the three girls made their way to the open front door of the bus and climbing on, spotted Emma and a couple of boarders from Whitby, sitting on the back seat that ran the full width of the bus. They all crowded on forming a noisy group at the rear of the bus. Then another long wait, it seemed to Emma, before the driver and conductress eventually reappeared and the bus finally pulled out of the station. They were off!

The conductress was slowly making her way up the aisle collecting the fares from the passengers and issuing them with tickets. The Middlesbrough girls had no problem stating their destination, but it was more difficult for Emma explaining that there was a signpost to Windrush where she wanted to get off although Emma knew she wasn't going to Windrush. The conductress, tall and beefy looking, with black hair tied in a bun, smiled at Emma.

'It's okay, love. I have a timetable here with all the stops on. I'll press the bell when it's your turn to get off and I'll give you a nod. Don't worry,' she added, reassuringly.

'Thank you,' replied Emma.

To pass the time away, the girls suggested playing games. 'Come on, who's going to start?' asked Maureen, the head boarder, sitting in the far corner of the seat. She was travelling to Middlesbrough.

'I'll give it a go,' offered Maria. Emma listened as the game progressed. One person gave clues about a film star and the others tried guess the name of the person described. There were a few wrong guesses and some laughter but generally the girls were quite quick to guess the correct name.

'You have a turn, Emma,' called Maria, who was sitting next to Maureen.

'I don't know any film stars.'

'You must know one or two, surely,' came a response.

'Everyone knows some film stars.'

'Not me,' thought Emma, racking her brains as to who she could describe. 'Right. The clue is, she is famous and is a ballet dancer.' The girls fired all sorts of questions and tried and tried but Emma kept shaking her head. They could not guess the correct answer.

'We give in. Who is it?'

'It's Petula Clark,' she stated, having remembered a picture with the name underneath, in a glossy magazine that Audrey lent her to read. There were peals of laughter.

'Oh, Emma. You are hopeless. She's a singer,' one of them stated, amidst the hilarity. Emma blushed, feeling most embarrassed and didn't reply. The game continued but Emma wasn't invited to participate again, much to her relief. She was happy just to listen, delighting in the knowledge that she'd soon be home.

After pulling into Whitby bus station, the driver steered the vehicle into its correct stand where further passengers were waiting to get on. A couple of the boarders said their goodbyes and dismounted along with a few other people. Whilst waiting for the driver to return, Emma gazed out of the window at the familiar surroundings, having been here many times. Whitby was the town where the Holmes family shopped, even though it was a ten-mile journey by bus to get there. When she'd turned ten years old, her parents trusted her for the first time, to travel alone on the bus to Whitby. She remembered that they'd given her a list of four items to buy and then to catch the bus home again. It was a daunting trip but soon, Emma grew in confidence and became accustomed to making the journey. She'd since done several trips alone on a Saturday or in the holidays when Tim and Martha were busy helping dad on the farm and mam stayed at home to see to the little ones. Sometimes Martha went with her, which was quite fun. They'd missed their bus once with dawdling along the harbour walkway eating an ice-cream, which mam said they could buy as a treat when they'd finished the shopping. They waited hours for the next bus and were given a good telling off when they finally arrived home.

Emma felt sick with excitement. A few more miles and she'd see her dad and mam again. She was longing for that moment. A couple of farmers, whom Emma recognised, climbed onto the bus and one of them looked over at Emma for a few seconds, before recognising her in her uniform.
'One o' Tom Holmes, a' ya?' Emma smiled and nodded.
'Gine yam, a' ya?' he continued.
'Yes, it's half-term,' she replied.
'Dus the like it, then?'
'Yes, thank you.' He told her he'd been visiting his wife in hospital and that she was on the mend.
'Tell ya dad, I was asking after 'im.' Emma nodded and smiled. The other girls were listening, finding the conversation fascinating.
'How do you understand him?' Maria asked, quietly. 'Most of the time, it sounds like a foreign language. What did he ask you?'
'It's easy. My dad talks like that. They all do around here. He asked me if I was going home and if I liked boarding school. He told me that his wife is in hospital but that she is getting better.' She was enjoying her moment.

Pressing her nose to the glass windowpane, Emma was watching the landmarks as the bus passed them by. She recognised familiar signposts, the farmhouses on the roadsides, the hedges and the turn-offs. She was in very familiar territory. Suddenly she jumped up.
'We're nearly there,' she voiced, excitedly.
'Where?' asked the girls, looking in the direction of her gaze.
'Over there across that moor, and look, there's my dad and our tractor. He's waiting for me.' She was beaming.
'Your stop coming up, lassie,' the cheerful conductress shouted to Emma from the front of the bus, but Emma was already hurrying down the aisle, brimming with delight whilst carrying her case carefully through the narrow passageway so as not to knock anyone with it.
'Bye. Have a good holiday,' the girls shouted. 'See you on

Tuesday.' The driver was pulling up at the Windrush signpost.

'There's your road to Windrush,' the conductress pointed out as Emma reached the front of the bus.

'Thank you, but I go the other way, over that track you can just make out, through the heather,' Emma replied, smiling broadly. The vehicle stopped and Emma, after turning around and waving to her companions, climbed down the steps and straight into her dad's arms.

Emma didn't want to let go. The tears started flowing as the built-up emotions of seven weeks bubbled over.

'Come on, lass,' said Tom. 'You're supposed to be pleased to see me, not sad,' and his daughter smiled through her tears. Letting go of Emma, Tom tied his binder band a little tighter around his button-less and ragged jacket and together they crossed the road. Tom climbed into his seat on the David Brown tractor which was parked on the rough grass. He started it up whilst Emma was joining him on the double seat from the opposite side and placing her suitcase on her knee, as the tractor began moving. It rumbled over the moor, down through the Muddy Hole, up the cart track with its bumps and holes on the other side and across more moor before Tom brought it to a halt at the top of the bank leading into Moorbeck valley. Emma jumped from the tractor and dragged the gate open for Tom, closing it afterwards before returning to her seat. This was home as she remembered. She loved being on the tractor with her dad and gave him a big grin as he glanced over to her. She repeated the process of opening and closing the gate at the bottom of the bank, following which, Tom steered the vehicle to the left approaching the farmhouse along the cobbles. He had barely brought it to a halt before Emma jumped off with her case and hurriedly made her way into the farmhouse.

'Hello,' she called, walking through the passage from the back kitchen to the family's living room. Mary met her as she came through the door and placing her arms around her daughter, hugged her tightly. Emma, on spying little Jacob who was occupied pushing a miniature toy car across the cement floor, released her hold on her mother and placing her case on the floor, bent down and picked him up. She kissed and cuddled him as he curled his arms tightly round her neck. Whilst holding him with one arm, she put her other arm around Amy, who was standing gazing up at her sister with a big grin on her little elfin face, her straight black fringe almost in her hazel-coloured eyes. Emma continued hugging them both. She was home. The tears were welling up again but happy tears this time. She couldn't believe just how much she'd missed them all. Mark walked in and gave his sister a cheeky grin. 'The same chubby Mark,' Emma thought. 'Aren't you going to give me a kiss, then?' she asked him, teasingly. Mark was more interested in something to eat.

'You'd better get that uniform off, Emma,' stated Mary. 'We don't want it getting torn or anything. That's a smart dress, better than the one you got from Mrs Raymons, although she meant kindly. I told you, didn't I, that we received a letter from Mother Monica explaining about it and she suggested we purchase another one. You got the second dress, didn't you,' Mary queried, 'as you never mentioned it in your letters?' Emma nodded.
'Sorry, Mam, I forgot to tell you. Mother Teresa gave me another one and told me you'd sent a cheque for it.'

Emma finally let go of the little ones, took off her coat and picking up her suitcase, began making her way towards the stairs' door.
'You're in the sitting room,' her mother said. 'We thought you and Martha would be okay in there whilst you're at home. We use it more as a bedroom, now you bairns are getting bigger. Take your coat with you and hang it behind the sitting room door. I think your clothes are on the bottom of your bed.' Emma nodded and crossed back over the passageway to the sitting room.
'Same old green distemper on the walls,' she thought, as she walked through the door. 'Cobwebs still hanging from the beams. Stuff shoved in corners. It's so unlike the tidy junior dormitory that I suppose I'm now used to. Still, it's home and I'm happy. Me and Martha will have a good chat tonight.' Emma quickly changed from her uniform into her familiar old clothes and went back into the farmhouse kitchen.

After the build-up of anticipation of the half-term holiday and the excitement of finally coming home wore off, Emma struggled somewhat with life on the farm, it being different to the living conditions of boarding school. She'd inevitably changed during those first seven weeks, as she'd slowly and with difficulty, adapted to a new way of life. She was used to electricity, flush toilets, running hot water from taps and meals all prepared. The silence and rigorous discipline, although so hard to take at first, was in total contrast to her home life, now seemingly disorganised. Going to the outside toilet was distasteful to her as the bucket slowly filled and was emptied only when Tom found a spare moment in his busy life. The torn-up Farmers Weekly paper was coarser compared with the toilet paper used at boarding school. It was a question of washing her hands under the cold water tap in the back kitchen or using a tin bowl with warm water in the living room, where the water slowly turned a murky grey with so many little hands using it, before being changed. Alternatively, either she or Martha took a large bowl of warm water into their downstairs bedroom for a proper wash, when wanting privacy.

The next morning, there was more uneasiness when Emma wandered down to the cowshed, after dressing. She entered the draughty building and slowly walked up the centre gangway, looking to chat with Martha. She spotted her halfway up the cowshed, perched on her three-legged stool, squirting milk into the bucket that was wedged between her black wellington boots. Martha, with her head half-buried into the side of the cow, was wearing her ragged old coat that she kept for this purpose along with her brown hand-knitted milking cap to protect her hair. Emma smiled when passing her thirteen-year-old brother Tim, also milking cows, whilst making her way to her sister. As Martha turned her head to speak to Emma, Emma gasped, as suddenly, a stream of warm milk found its mark on her face and trickled down her chin, only for a second, before Tom, grinning widely, redirected the milk back into his bucket. When younger, the children found this hilarious as he played his little prank on them but this time, Emma was not amused.
'It's not funny, Dad,' she exclaimed, wiping her face with the back of her sleeve.

Emma had tried hard at practising her vowel sounds and speech after having the elocution lessons and this was evident in her conversations with her peer group. Although she did not care much for the lessons, Emma was happy to do attend them, having been teased at school on her strange pronunciation of many words. Her tutor told her that there was a marked improvement even over the space of a few weeks as Emma was determined not to be laughed at again about her local accent. This now backfired at home. 'It's not funny, dad,' retorted Tom, mimicking her and putting on a posh voice instead of his usual broad Yorkshire accent. Emma was embarrassed and confused, because, having learnt to speak more correctly like her peer group at school, she was finding that equally, she was speaking differently from her family at home. *It's not funny, dad,* said in a very posh voice, became a joke to be tossed around the family, much to everyone's amusement.

Emma, mulling over this incident throughout the short half-term at home, was becoming conscious of just how broad in speech her parents were, something that was without meaning to her before her attendance at the grammar school. The contrast between life on the farm and her experience at boarding school was becoming evident to Emma and she was beginning to realise that her life at Bankside farm would not be quite the same again. Mary, who'd lived in a another part of the country before coming to Whitby and meeting Tom, knew that when Emma was older, she would realise that people came from all walks of life with a variety of different accents and it just wasn't that important, but she could see that Emma was feeling this deeply during her first return home after seven weeks in a different environment. Mary tried to deflect the merriment that was at Emma's expense when in the farmhouse kitchen as she was acutely aware of Emma's discomfort.

Despite these new difficulties for Emma, she enjoyed her four days at home even if a little strained at times trying to bridge a seven-week break in relationships with her brothers and sisters. When the time came so quickly for her to return to boarding school, she was sorry to leave the home security and love of her family. She felt a weight at the pit of her stomach and a pull on her heart strings as she hugged her mam goodbye whilst fighting the tears that sprung to her eyes. Tom interrupted his busy workload on the farm to take her on the tractor to the bus stop near the turn-off to Windrush. He watched his daughter struggle with tears as she opened and closed the gates on the way. When almost at the end of the cart track, he pulled up for Emma to dismount and make her way across the road to the bus stop but not before he himself climbed down and hugged her. He then waited on his tractor parked on the moor until the red bus appeared and came to a halt.

After getting onto the bus, Emma stood inside the aisle and gave her dad one last wave before moving along to where she spotted a couple of boarders. She squeezed into an empty seat and nursing her small case, tried to compose herself as she felt so emotional, mentally adjusting to the separation from her family. After the bus journey, Emma, putting herself into forward gear to face another period of weeks before she would see her family again, was very subdued as she walked through the streets of Scarborough, trailing behind the girls in front who were chattering continuously about their short holiday.

When Emma entered the boarders' room, she spied Faith talking to Audrey. As the two girls both travelled by train from the same town, they made the journey back to school together and immediately on seeing Emma, they waved her over.
'Did you enjoy your holiday?' questioned Faith. Emma nodded, still struggling with the separation from her family.
'It was lovely seeing Martha and the rest of them. I got loads of hugs.'
'I've brought a book to lend you,' said Audrey. 'Faith told me how much you like reading. I always bring two or three back with me. When you've finished with it, let me know and I'll lend you another.'
'Oh, thanks, Audrey.' Emma's eyes lit up. She skimmed through the write-up on the back cover. It was a school mystery story. 'That's great,' Emma enthused. 'Thank you so much.'
'It's okay,' replied Audrey, pleased that she could bring a

smile to Emma's face, having noticed how downcast she
appeared when entering the boarders' room.

Faith and Audrey continued their conversation about the
pictures they'd been to at their local cinema. Emma listened,
again feeling on the outside. She fingered the book she was
holding, looking forward to starting it.
'Maybe tonight,' she thought, 'when I'm in bed although
lights go out at nine but maybe I'll have time for a little read.'
Her spirits lifted. 'Did you see Audrey over the holidays?'
Emma asked Faith, after Audrey wandered off to speak to
Polly who'd entered the room.
'Yes, I bumped into her when walking to the picture house. I
was on my own as my mam was working and my sister was
out with her boyfriend. Afterwards she invited me to her
home. Like I told you, she lives in a flat above a shop that
her parents own. It's a bigger and smarter place than ours.
Now that I've seen hers, I can't imagine asking her back to
mine. Ours is cramped and scruffy.' She looked ruefully at
Emma for a moment before changing the subject.
'Maybe she's a bit like me,' pondered Emma, later. 'Not
much money and all that.'

Emma knew that every day in the convent chapel, Mass was
celebrated by a priest from the local church, but apart from
Sundays, boarders were only obliged to attend on Tuesdays
and Thursdays. In a conversation with Maria one evening,
she discovered that if she wanted, she could go on the other
days provided she asked the supervising nun in the
dormitory for an early morning call.
'You strip your bed before you go,' said Maria, 'and make it
when you return, whilst the others are getting dressed.
Another thing is that you don't need to go to morning prayers
if you've been to Mass.'
'Does that mean, whilst the rest go to chapel after breakfast
and then to the dormitories to make their beds, I have free
time?' Maria nodded.

Emma thought about this and decided to give it a go, as she
welcomed the idea of doing something different. By the end
of the week and having been to early morning Mass three
times without the other boarders, she found that she enjoyed

the break from the rigorous discipline of routine, as well as having a little personal time to herself. 'Maybe not the ideal reasons for going to Mass,' she thought, but it suited her. Also, with no-one around in the early hours, Emma took the stairs three at a time as she loved running down the broad, large stairs, unlike hers at home which were narrow and much steeper. At first, she sometimes whistled, a habit she'd acquired at home on the farm, until overheard one day by a nun.

'Don't you know that it makes Our Lady blush to hear you whistle,' the nun stated. Emma didn't, but was also told that it was unladylike too and she stopped doing it.

'I guess they're trying to make a lady out of me,' thought Emma, 'whatever that means.'

Emma recalled the first time she requested an early morning call, even though she felt embarrassed at asking the nun, as she wasn't keen on anyone knowing. She'd quickly and quietly washed at the sink and dressed before creeping out of the dormitory and making her way down the flights of stairs to the chapel. It was then she discovered one or two more boarders were doing likewise, including Maria. Emma wasn't sure where to sit but she'd ventured down the aisle to a bench near the front of the chapel. At the distribution of Holy Communion, she remembered hesitating about when to approach the altar rails. There seemed to be so many nuns coming and coming. When she'd decided she'd waited long enough, she slipped in among them and knelt amidst a row of nuns. A little later, she saw Maria and another boarder join the end of the line, following the nuns. It was another embarrassing moment for Emma when Maria pointed out, after Mass, that they must wait until all the nuns have taken Communion before they approach the rails.

'I must have stood out like a sore thumb,' thought Emma, blushing at the thought of it.

'Did you sell many of those raffle books at half-term?' asked Faith, one evening at recreation, later in the term. 'You took loads of them.' The school was having a grand raffle to be drawn at the end of term. The day girls collected the raffle books over the weeks to try and sell them, but for the boarders, half-term at home was the only time available.

Emma took many books home as she knew that her parents would be very supportive. Her dad, when he'd gone to Whitby on the Saturday of half-term, had taken some, as he always called in The Wellington for a pint or two before getting the bus home. He'd sold quite a number.

Mary carried plenty in her handbag to church on the Sunday. When the women congregated outside after Mass, Mary explained about the fundraising and they were most happy to purchase some. The parishioners were very generous. She even approached Mrs Stoutly, at The General Dealers, after church, when she went to buy The Farmers Weekly and a few sweets for the children. Mr Stoutly expressed his interest in Emma's progress and both were happy to purchase raffle books, no doubt partly because Mary and Tom were good customers each Sunday.

Tom, meanwhile, went into the Hunters Lodge for his usual pint after Mass. He handed around the books of tickets to his mates, on the quiet insistence from Mary that he must take them as the fellows would be happy to buy, she thought. She was right. Jack Netherfield was the first to pull out a note from his jacket pocket and buy half a dozen books. Following this example, the other men were equally as forthcoming with their money as the parishioners at church and Tom quickly pocketed the stubs with the cash before having his usual game of dominoes. This was a social event for many farmers, whilst wives either joined them or waited outside, as in Mary's case, with children. It was only a quick game and the children enjoyed their drink of lemonade.

Emma was delighted when Mary handed her the money and stubs to take back to school.

'Mam, you've done great,' Emma gushed, so happy to be taking all the sold books back.

'Such good prizes,' said Mary. 'People were impressed with the list of prizes especially the star prize, a choice of a bicycle, or the equivalent in cash. That's a great prize. Your dad told me how generous Jack Netherfield was. He's okay with your dad now. He doesn't drink like he did when he was ill. He was ill, you know.' Emma nodded, not quite sure about what the illness was that made him drink too much alcohol but was glad they were all friends.

In answer to Faith's question, Emma nodded her head. 'My mam and dad sold them. When I handed them in to Mother Monica, she told me to go and see Mother Margaret, but I haven't been yet.' It was at the last assembly before half-term that Mother Monica announced that anyone selling more than twelve books could collect a small gift from Mother Margaret's office. She was the Reverend Mother Superior and in overall charge of all the nuns at the convent. Her small office was situated in the main corridor of the building near to the main doors. Emma had never been inside her office. Mother Margaret was a very tall, slim woman with a long, angular face, pointed features, and usually wore narrow-rimmed spectacles. She looked quite forbidding to Emma when the nun was pointed out to her in chapel, by Maria, at an early morning weekday Mass.

'Why don't you go now,' stated Faith. 'Just explain to Mother Catherine that Mother Monica told you to go. She'll be okay about it. I'll go with you if you like and wait outside while you go in.' Mother Catherine was on duty supervising the boarders at recreation. So very timidly, Emma asked permission and Mother Catherine said it was okay but to come straight back afterwards. She gave permission for Faith to go with her. They made their way past the form rooms to the main corridor and Emma gently knocked on the door of the office.

'Come in,' called a clear high-pitched voice.
'You'll be fine,' whispered Faith. Emma turned the knob and pushed open the door and stepped inside, leaving the door slightly ajar.
'Yes?' questioned the nun from behind her desk and peering over her spectacles at this dark-haired young girl. 'What can I do for you?'
'Mother Monica told me to come as I've sold more than twelve books of raffle tickets and I think I get a small gift. I have asked permission to leave recreation, from Mother Catherine.' Emma floundered, not knowing what else to say and feeling in awe of this nun. Mother Margaret studied the little girl.
'I don't think we've met except maybe at your interview. What is your name?'

'I'm Emma Holmes.'

'Who sold the tickets for you?' the nun gently enquired. 'Was it at half-term?'

'Yes. I took them home and my mam sold them at church on the Sunday and my dad sold them in the pub at Whitby where he goes, after doing the shopping. He sold some in the pub at Windrush as well. That's where he has a pint with the farmers after Mass on Sundays.' Mother Margaret smiled at this lengthy and somewhat unusual but very honest reply.

'You tell your parents that we are most grateful for their support. They have done well. You live on a farm, do you?' Emma nodded.

'It's called Bankside in Moorbeck.' Mother Catherine smiled again.

'And you have brothers and sisters, do you?'

'There's five at home. Two older than me and three younger ones.'

'You're happy here, are you Emma? I imagine it's quite different for you.'

'It's all right, thank you,' Emma replied without further explanation, watching Mother Margaret opening a drawer and taking out array of oddments that she placed on her desktop, after moving aside some papers to make space for them.

'You may choose one,' she invited Emma, her hand gesturing towards the objects.

Emma scanned them but couldn't see much of interest. She spotted a six-inch bronze statue of Jesus and although it didn't look new, as it had been at some stage painted blue and the colour was wearing off in places, Emma thought she could stand it on her locker beside her bed. Most of the boarders had ornaments or photos on their locker tops but she didn't have anything.

'I'll have something to display now,' she thought. 'I'll take this, thank you,' she said politely to the nun, picking up the statue, before turning around and quietly leaving the room, closing the door behind her. She was glad to get that over with.

'Well?' said Faith, as they began walking back to the hall.

'It was fine. She was nice to me. I got this as I didn't know what to pick,' Emma replied, revealing the small statue from her curled fingers. Faith smiled as they reached the hall door just in time to hear Mother Catherine clap her hands for everyone to stop talking and line up to go to the dormitories.

After arriving in the dormitory with her little statue, Emma placed it on her locker and was quite pleased to have something on view like the other girls. As it was not an obligatory Mass, the following day, she'd intended, on her way to bed, to ask for an early morning call. She realised that she forgotten and went back down the corridor to the main entrance to the dormitory where she knew the nun would be seated at her small table. The cold mornings didn't stop Emma rising early, but she found her thin eiderdown plus two blankets were not enough to keep her warm at night. Whilst asking Mother Teresa for a wake-up call, she finally plucked up the courage to ask her about the possibility of borrowing a blanket.
'I am cold in bed at night,' she explained. 'I wonder if there is a blanket I could borrow, please.' She knew that there were spare blankets at the bottom of the communal wardrobe at the end of their dormitory.
'Of course, Emma. I'll come with you to get one.' They walked back to the junior dormitory together and over to the wardrobe where Mother Teresa took out an old thin grey blanket and handed it to Emma. 'There you are. Another layer will help.'
'Thank you,' replied Emma, taking the folded blanket. 'The nun was right,' she thought later when snuggled up in bed. The blanket, although thin, was larger than her covers and she found that by tucking it in all round her bed, it held all her covers in place making it much warmer for her.

Once established back into the routine at boarding school, Emma was reasonably happy with her studies and the easy life compared with home and farm jobs. She relished the bath times especially.
'The joy of running hot water,' she thought, 'plus having heating throughout the large building and not having to huddle around a coal fire like we do at home for warmth when the colder nights begin.' Emma often spent the evening recreation hugging a radiator and reading her book. Sometimes Maria joined her, also reading. Emma

remembered that Maria told her one morning when they caught each other on the stairs going to early Mass that she was the eldest of a large family. She imagined that Maria probably appreciated the opportunity for a quiet read.

Emma still yearned for cuddles from her family and either playing cards with her mam and dad and Tim and Martha in the evenings or joining in the singsongs with the family. She missed the open fields and the walks to the wood where they climbed the trees and played hide and seek in the tall bracken. 'Never mind,' she thought. 'It will soon be Christmas holidays.' She mentally consoled herself by listing other advantages that she was growing accustomed to having, such as the flush toilets, ready cooked meals even though rather meagre at times, plus the pleasant weekend walks.

It was towards the end of the term that Emma made a second visit to the Reverend Mother's office and this time, it was a very pleasurable visit. The day in question started with the whole school being assembled in the hall shortly before Christmas. All lay staff and teaching nuns were on the stage when Mother Margaret joined them to oversee the drawing of the Christmas raffle. The first ticket drawn was for the star prize. Mother Margaret beckoned one of the day girls at the very front of the hall to come onto the stage and pull one out from the large bag full of folded raffle tickets. Hundreds of pairs of eyes, every girl in the hall, were watching and waiting. The young pupil dug deeply into the bag and handed a folded ticket to the nun, before returning to her place.

There was complete silence as Mother Margaret unfolded the ticket and scrutinised it before smiling and showing it to the nuns on each side of her. They too smiled. There was a slight pause.
'The name of the winner for the star prize,' called out Mother Margaret, reading from the ticket stub, 'is Emma Holmes, Bankside Farm, Moorbeck, Windrush, Whitby.' The whole assembly clapped. The girls at the front of the hall around Emma were not only clapping but cheering also and those who could reach her were slapping her on the back. Emma

was flabbergasted and didn't know what to do. She half-moved forward and then stood up before sitting down again. She didn't know if she was supposed to go onto the stage or just stay put. She could see all the staff including the nuns smiling and looking in her direction.

'It's me,' she thought. 'It's me. I've won first prize.' The noise abated. The draw continued but Emma's mind was in a whirl and she could no longer concentrate on what was going on.

It was later in the morning when Emma made her way to the office of Mother Margaret to ask about the prize. She was nervous about going but Faith and Audrey encouraged her to go and even accompanied her, as it was break time. Emma knocked on the door with trepidation and after being called to enter, she opened the door and went inside, closing it after herself, leaving the other two waiting outside.

'It's me, again,' she said anxiously, looking at Mother Margaret who was busy writing at her desk. 'I've come about the raffle prize.'

'Hello, Emma. Congratulations. Aren't you a lucky girl,' stated Mother Margaret, smiling at her. 'Would you like the bicycle, or would you prefer to have the money?' she queried.

'Oh, the money, please,' replied Emma, without any hesitation. She'd never owned a bike and hadn't learnt to ride. The bumpy cart tracks in Moorbeck were not ideal for bicycle riding. Choosing a bicycle didn't mean much to her but taking the money certainly did. She was anticipating the pleasure it would give her to hand the money over to her parents to help them at Christmas time. 'They sold all the tickets anyway,' she reasoned to herself. 'They could have the money.' Mother Margaret wrote out the cheque for twelve pounds five shillings and handed it to Emma.

'There you are. Take it to Mother Monica's office and ask her to place it in your purse until we break up. Only a few more days now. I hope you and your family have a lovely Christmas.' Emma whispered her thanks, still in awe of this high-ranking nun, but with her face glowing, thinking of the lovely surprise for her parents.

'Did you choose the bike, then?' asked Audrey, as Emma joined the two girls still waiting for her outside the door.

Emma shook her head. 'Why didn't you?' Audrey questioned, thinking how lovely a brand-new bicycle would be, but then, as Emma knew, Audrey lived in a market town with plenty of roads to cycle along. She shrugged her shoulders but didn't reply. She knew that Audrey was an only child and judging by the frequent parcels she received and the style of her clothes that she changed into, after lessons, thought that she wouldn't understand what it was like to be poor. Emma didn't feel like explaining to her how much the money would mean to her own parents.

On the last evening before breaking up for the Christmas holidays, the girls were in the boarders' room as usual, restless because of having no homework. Mother Catherine, sitting quietly at her table, chose to ignore the whisperings that were all around her.
'It is the last evening after all,' she thought. 'A little relaxation of the rules won't do any harm,' she reasoned to herself. She'd only been seated a few minutes when the door opened. Mother Monica walked in. The whisperings ceased. She walked over to the table and spoke quietly to Mother Catherine who nodded before standing up and leaving the room. Mother Monica placed several folders on the table adding to the pile already there, before sitting down. Only then, did Emma realise that what looked like folders were report books.
'Our school reports,' she thought. 'Now what happens.'

'Good evening, girls,' greeted Mother Monica.
'Good evening, Mother,' came a chorus of voices.
'As most of you know but for the benefit of the new boarders, this is customary on the last evening of each term. I will read out the name and position gained in their Form before handing the report to the pupil in question. Maybe a few comments too if I deem it necessary,' she added, smiling across the room. She began with year one and then to year two when Polly's name was called and following hers, one by one, the names of the other boarders in her Form. Emma listened intently as she expected it would be their turn next. It was. Audrey was placed fourth and Faith came seventh. Mother Monica took the next report from the large stack and opened it and glanced across at Emma.

'Emma Holmes,' Mother Monica read out. 'Well done. You have come first in your Form. This is an excellent report with all comments very affirming of your hard work and diligent approach to your studies.' Emma stood up and walked to the table to take her report from the nun. She was delighted. Another surprise for her mam and dad. She knew they would be so pleased with her.

It was a bit tedious waiting for Mother Monica to finish giving out the report books, Emma thought, but she didn't really mind as she felt so happy.
'And now,' Mother Monica stated, after handing out the last report, 'you may go and collect your cases from the attic, in an orderly fashion, girls, please. There is a little time left to pack, before supper. Take your report with you and don't forget to have your parent or guardian sign it before returning it to my office when you arrive back in January.' Mother Monica stood and beckoned Maureen to lead the girls out of the room.

The following afternoon, Emma was stepping off the bus again at the Windrush stop. It was raining, cold and windy. The moors looked desolate and grey. After the hustle and bustle of the last few days at boarding school, she was tired but looking forward to her Christmas holiday. She slowly made her way, carrying her heavy case, along the muddy wet potholed cart track with the rain sleeting across the moor, forming a murky shadowy view across the bleak countryside. She was told by her mam in her last letter that if Tom wasn't waiting for her at the bus stop, to start walking home. He would come if he could. Eventually Emma could faintly hear a low rumble, realising, as it increased in volume, that it was the noise of the tractor that she could hear. She eventually spied it in the distance looming ever closer.

Tom, having decided to make time to pick up his daughter, found that his tractor wouldn't start. Time and time again, he swung the handle around, but it just wouldn't kick in. He eventually succeeded. On driving through the Muddy Hole, he realised why it had such a name as water and mud were flying everywhere from the tractor wheels. The cart track in this dip was a sludgy mess of water, stones and mud. He finally met with Emma at the top of the other side of Muddy Hole. She waited whilst he turned his tractor around on the heather and pulled up beside her.

'Sorry I'm late. The tractor wouldn't start.' Emma smiled at her dad as she put her suitcase into the link-box and climbed onto the tractor, the water running down her face and dripping from the end of her nose. She couldn't contain her good news any longer.

'Dad, I've got a lovely surprise. I've come top of my Form and I won the star prize in the raffle and I chose the money instead of a bike. Remember, all those books you and mam sold. Well, I've got a cheque for twelve pounds five shillings for you.' Tom put one arm around his daughter, steering with the other one whilst the rain was lashing down. His daughter had made it. Top of the Form. He was proud of her and delighted with the money as things were so tight especially at Christmas time.

'We'll have a lovely Christmas, lass, but first, we'll get you home and out of those wet clothes.' They sat side by side on the double seat. All the hard work and sacrificing was paying off, Tom thought. He couldn't wait to tell Mary.

Spring to Summer 1952

The spring term at the boarding school passed uneventfully for Emma. She knuckled down with her studies and learnt to accept the routine of discipline without being too upset. Pangs of homesickness were less frequent. Mary continued to write her weekly letter, albeit often quite short. Sometimes, a letter arrived from Martha, a substitute for Mary's. Emma found Martha's letters to be interesting and enjoyable as they were more detailed about goings-on at Bankside and this helped her to feel connected to the life on the farm even though it was in total contrast to her boarding school routine. Faith and Emma were slowly developing a mutual friendship that helped in cushioning Emma's times of sadness.

It was the summer school term that brought new trials for Emma. Swimming lessons were added to the curriculum. Most of the girls in her form could swim, either having had access to local swimming baths or having been taken regularly to a swimming pool further afield by their parents. Emma had never been to a swimming pool. Her only access to the possibility of swimming was when Mary and her cousin-in-law on the farm across the valley in Moorbeck made the annual trip with their children to the nearest beach for a day out. Emma was always delighted with these trips and loved to venture out to sea as far as she dared, but she could not swim. She found the thoughts of the swimming pool sessions very daunting. She was most apprehensive.

'Will you wait for me please,' she asked Faith, 'as I've never been to the baths before.'
'Never?' exclaimed Faith, in amazement. She found this hard to believe as she was a regular swimmer at the local baths in Bartown, as was Audrey. On arriving at the indoor swimming pool, Faith showed Emma what to do.
'You take one of these wire holders in which you place your clothes when you change into your swimming costume. You keep the disc with the number on so that you can reclaim your clothes when we return to the dressing area after our swimming lesson. I can't believe you've never been swimming before.'

'Well, I haven't,' said Emma, defensively. 'We go to the sands once a year and I bathe in the sea, but I can't swim.'

Having handed over her clothes, Emma followed Faith to the pool itself. Immediately she noticed that the level of noise was almost deafening. Girls were shouting, squealing and laughing. There were girls diving in at the far end and swimming the full length of the pool. She watched others climb to the top of the water chute, coming down at great speed, sending splashes of water flying in all directions as they hit the water before disappearing under it. They reappeared on the surface, gasping for breath. Some girls were ducking and diving and pulling each other under with lots of splashing and hilarity. It was second nature to most of them, this playful lesson in the pool and she envied their total lack of fear.

The PE teacher spotted Emma and waved her over to the far edge of the pool at the shallow end, to stand alongside two other rather nervous looking girls. Mrs Carruthers was short and stocky with a square face and clipped, grey hair. She doesn't look like a PE teacher, thought Emma, but nevertheless, she found Mrs Carruthers to be fair and kind, even if a little brusque at times when she took them for indoor gymnastics and exercises. She'd never belittled Emma when she couldn't do the leg stretches at the bars in the big hall. Those who went to ballet were very graceful and raised their legs high as a ballerina would. Emma struggled with that but came into her own when climbing the ropes dangling from the high ceiling at one end of the hall. Not many of the girls could achieve more than a few over hands before they were tired, whereas Emma, after two or three attempts, managed to reach the top of the rope and then gingerly, hand over hand, slowly made her way down, feeling very pleased with herself. She also moved swiftly like a monkey across the climbing bars when they had a chasing game.
'All the hard work at home has given me muscles and strength,' she mused, smiling to herself, 'and now I know what these wooden bars are for.'

The teacher's voice penetrated her thoughts and brought

Emma back to the present.

'I take it that you can't swim either?'

'No, I can't. This is my very first visit to a swimming pool,' Emma responded, almost shamefully. The teacher sensed her fearfulness.

'We'll take it gently today. Lower yourselves into the water and get a feel of it. Walk into the deeper water as far as you feel comfortable. We won't start the swimming lessons today. It's important you feel confident in the water first.' Emma climbed gently down the steps, slowly immersing herself to waist level and discovered that the water was pleasantly warm. She floundered around in two feet of water, feeling her feet on the floor of the pool. Slowly, Emma moved her body into slightly deeper water and felt comfortable until she sensed that her feet no longer seemed to be standing on a solid surface. She quickly manoeuvred around and made her way back to safer waters. Faith came swimming across the pool, pulling herself to her feet in front of Emma. She was totally at ease in the water.

'Come and have a go down the chute,' she invited Emma. 'It's shallow at the bottom. It doesn't matter if you can't swim. You can't drown in three feet of water.' Emma hesitated. 'I think I'll wait until next week. Maybe I'll be a little more confident then.' Faith smiled and swam back out into the deep water.

'If only…,' thought Emma.

'Well, girls. I think we will try a little breaststroke today,' said the teacher, the following week, already standing in the pool with the non-swimmers at the shallow end. 'Hold onto the bar and push your legs out so,' she demonstrated. After several times carrying out this manoeuvre, Emma found it quite easy and she was able to stretch her legs well out across the water. 'Now turn around and we'll practise arm movements,' instructed the teacher. This seemed simple enough to Emma. 'Co-ordinating these movements is slightly more difficult,' continued the teacher, 'but we'll try that next week. Just keep practising or testing the deeper waters.'

On the third visit to the pool, Emma decided she would have a go down the chute. She hauled her seemingly heavy body up over the edge of the pool, dragging herself out and walking around to the top of the chute, where she climbed on. She then almost panicked. It looked so far down to the water. Audrey spotted her.

'Come on,' she called, from below.

'I daren't.'

'Oh, come on. Don't chicken out,' Audrey retorted. A small group of girls were looking on with interest, splashing around at the bottom of the chute.

'Come on. Don't be a coward,' one called out.

'Yes, come on, scaredy, scaredy,' shouted another. Emma was becoming angry, not liking this catcalling.

'Sticks and stones may hurt my bones but calling names won't hurt me,' she chanted back at them. Then, with her hands holding tightly to the sides of the chute, she gingerly edged her way carefully down the slope. Inch by inch, she moved her body, making very slow progress whilst ignoring the laughter of the girls below as they watched her efforts. When there was only a couple of feet left at the end of the chute, she removed her hands and slid into the water with hardly a splash. Her peer group lost interest and returned to swim more lengths. Emma, determined to overcome her fears, climbed out of the pool and went back to the top of the chute. This time, although slowly edging her way down as before, she let go a little further away from the bottom of the chute. It was becoming easier. Over and over, she repeated this performance improving each time until she heard the whistle signalling the end of the lesson. On her last attempt, sitting at the top of the chute, she let go of the handrails and slid down at top speed into the water, gulping for breath as she resurfaced, but feeling a great thrill of satisfaction. She was happy.

It was many weeks before Emma managed to swim a few strokes in the shallow end of the pool, her feet slowly sinking to the bottom each time she tried, but she loved splashing around and doing a doggy paddle. The chute held no fear either nor did sliding off it at speed into the water, enjoying the whoosh of the waves almost engulfing her.

'Maybe one day, I will manage to swim a width and possibly dare to try a length,' she thought, unconvinced that this would happen soon. Emma was only happy if her feet could feel the bottom of the pool. The teacher then discussed learning to dive but Emma was reluctant, not liking it when her face went under water.

'I think I'll leave that for next year,' she told herself, putting off what, to her, seemed like an unnecessary ordeal.

During the warm summer days of late June and early July, the weekend long walks were a joy. One Saturday, some of the older boarders were asked to help in the refectory to prepare food for a picnic. This entailed slicing and filling dozens and dozens of bread buns which were placed in small baskets, covered with cloths and left in the refectory to be collected by the girls. It was time-consuming providing enough buns for thirty to forty of them and the younger ones in the boarders' room were becoming impatient, eager to set off.

'I think that will do,' commented Maureen who was overseeing the preparation and counting the number of baskets. 'I'll go and tell Mother that we're ready. It's a good job we don't do this too often but thank you for all your hard work.'

Arriving at Marine Drive with the magnificent views stretching far out over the sea, the girls broke rank and strolled side by side or in groups, enjoying the warmth of the sun and the freedom to saunter. On reaching the far end, they began walking towards a cove where there were plenty of large rocks to sit on. Some of the younger ones, immediately they arrived, removed their socks and shoes and went running across the wide expanse of sand to the sea, a long way off as the tide was going out.

'Race you,' Audrey shouted gleefully to Emma. They pelted down to the water's edge and along the rippled sand, puffing and panting and laughing. Coming to a halt, they gingerly tested the waters with their toes.

'What a beautiful blue sky,' said Emma, gazing upwards. 'It reminds me of home. We have days like this on the farm, you know, when we paddle in the beck,' she explained to Audrey, as they sauntered back to the group.

The summer term ticked by. Exams were looming on the horizon. Emma was top of her Form again at Easter, but she didn't think she would retain that position at the end of the year. She knew that some of the girls were trying extra hard as they were bent on putting her down a few notches. Audrey, as nice as she was to Emma, was one of those determined to improve her position and overtake her. After the ordeal of the exams, excitement was building up again at the approaching end of term. Long summer holidays were being anticipated. Emma was looking forward to the thrill of packing, of seeing all the suitcases piled up ready to be carried by willing hands. Although the farewells and breakups were almost sad at each holiday break for the boarders, she guessed that the eager anticipation of the many weeks of freedom would far outweigh them, this time.

The night before the mass exodus at the end of the summer term, was the usual ritual of reports being handed out in the boarders' room. Emma's hard work paid off. She'd made fourth position overall which she was happy with. Audrey was delighted to have overtaken her, but Emma didn't care. She acknowledged to herself that she couldn't stay at the top all the time. She knew her parents would be delighted with her highly satisfactory report. She might not have achieved *Excellent* for conduct, but she was happy with *Very Good*. Faith improved her position by one place and was pleased with herself.

On this last evening of the school year, after supper, the boarders had a tradition of a singsong instead of the usual recreation. They were cramped together in the music room because the large assembly hall was unavailable. Alongside some well-known songs, crazy songs were sung, composed of exaggerated descriptions relating to the conditions of boarding school life and these were chanted in schoolgirl fashion. Emma, with Faith sitting beside her, soon caught on and joined in with this frivolous singing.

No more Latin, no more French. No more sitting on a hard school bench.
No more going through chapel door coming out with knees damn sore.
No more spiders in my bath, trying hard to make me laugh.
No more beetles in my tea, making googly eyes at me.

The rhymes continued amidst smiles and giggles. Mother Teresa, on duty tonight, turned a blind eye and was even

smiling quietly at this uproarious singing that increased in volume as the girls were coming to the end of recreation time. They finished with an old favourite that included the repeated rendition:
Wherever I may wander, wherever I may roam, there's no place like home, there's no place like home.

As the boarders were finishing this song, the atmosphere changed. The singing began to fade away as some of the girls were struggling with their emotions. Faith whispered to Emma.
'I think it's affecting some of the oldest ones. They look as if they might cry. Can you see, over in the corner towards the back of the room?' Emma glanced across and nodded. Emma and Faith were quite amazed, at the end of the singsong, at the reaction of some pupils who were leaving permanently. One or two older boarders who were not coming back, were shedding a tear or two but one girl broke down completely and sobbed. It dawned on Emma that these girls had spent the best part of the last five to seven years together, living through the highs and lows of growing up. She didn't feel anything towards these older girls as she hardly knew them. She couldn't imagine being like that, when she finally left.

As the girls streamed out of the music room, even apart from the tearful ones, others were quite subdued. It was a longer walk than usual, as the music room was almost at the furthest end of the building away from the boarders' area. Joanne caught up with Emma as they turned into the next corridor.
'You look deep in thought. Anything the matter?' she enquired, kindly.
'I was thinking about those girls who are leaving and how upset some of them were. I don't understand it. I love going home to Bankside.'
'Even though the girls might consider boarding school difficult with its discipline, especially during the later teen years, it's the close bonds that are formed,' Joanne replied, quietly. 'You see, Emma, this place with all its goings on, in fact, has been their home and in some instances, has given a sense of security and normality to those whose home lives

are disjointed and unpredictable. It's almost a protection, shielding some of the girls from what might have been a more traumatic teenage life. It's been a very structured and stable life for them here.'
'I never thought of it like that.'
'Well, my mother has explained a few things to me about it,' responded Joanne. 'Being a teacher herself, she hears stuff that maybe some parents aren't aware of. It's quite nostalgic for some boarders and they struggle with leaving for good and having to face a big wide world, out there.'

The girls whispered amongst themselves whilst climbing the flights of stairs to the dormitory, some walking two or three abreast. Mother Teresa following behind, making no attempt to exert the rules. She could see that some of the girls were upset.
'It is the last night here for some weeks,' she reasoned. 'What harm was there, in them having a last little chat together.' She also chose to ignore rules being broken in the junior dormitory as the girls were too excited to sleep. Whispering continued for quite some time. Faith sneaked out of bed and crept across to Emma's and leaning towards her bed, spoke very quietly to her.
'In case, I don't have time tomorrow or don't catch you before you leave, I hope you have a wonderful summer holiday. I'll be thinking of you when I'm alone at the swimming baths or pictures.' Emma smiled.
'Maybe one day, you could come with me and have a few days at Bankside. I might discuss it with mam and dad.' Faith's light blue eyes shone in the darkness.
'I'd love that,' she whispered, adding, 'sleep well,' before padding back to her own bed. Emma finally fell asleep wondering if she should have said that.
'What about having no bathroom or hot water,' she'd thought. 'What would Faith make of Emma's home life? The little ones? It was noisy at times. She'd have to share a bed. I'll have a think when I get home.'

One morning, a few days into her holiday, Emma was eyeing the messy, overcrowded farmhouse kitchen.
'Some things never change,' she thought, 'and I don't know what Faith would make of all this.' She sighed. She was

comparing it with the spaciousness of the convent boarding school rooms. Here in the kitchen, small cars, wooden bricks, the stray crayon, oddments of clothing and old washed-out cushions were all jumbled on the chairs, on the cement floor and on the clip mat in front of the fire. The ash in the fireplace was accumulating and needed removing. Two-year-old Jacob was whizzing around the room in his bare feet but going as fast as his little legs would take him, holding a toy airplane in his chubby fingers whilst making a humming noise. Flies were buzzing about even though there was a long sticky fly catcher hanging from the ceiling covered with dead and dying flies. Amy was seated at the table, wading her way through a bowl of cornflakes, whilst Mark was trying to make himself a cup of tea.

'Here, let me do that for you, Mark. Aren't you a bit little to be using that kettle?'

'I am nine, now, you know. Amy can't but she's only six. Mam lets me if I'm careful,' he replied, adeptly pouring boiling water into his cup. Bedroom floors were littered too, she'd noticed yesterday when she'd paid a visit upstairs to help Amy search for her cardigan. She was accustomed to the orderliness of boarding school life and was finding it difficult adjusting to the contrasting experience of home life.

Mary walked in with a jug full of milk, fresh and warm, straight from the milking done this morning.

'Oh, you're up, Emma. Put the kettle on again and then can you see to Jacob's shoes for him please. Dad and Martha and Tim are on their way in for breakfast. Jacob, just slow down a bit, there's a good lad,' she added, almost in collision with him with the milk jug still in her hand. Jacob grinned and slowed to a toddle.

'Okay,' replied Emma, tidying the table and putting more cups out for the workers after putting the kettle on the ring above the coal fire. She turned to catch Jacob who delighted in running from her.

'Catch me, catch me,' he yelled excitedly, before trying to escape through the kitchen door, opened by his fourteen-year-old brother. Tim was growing tall, but gangly, his arms and legs being out of proportion to his torso. He needed a shave of the sparsely growing hairs on his top lip.

'Gotcha,' he said, as he scooped Jacob into his arms and

handed him to Emma. 'Shoes on!'

Alongside the familiarity of sameness in her home, there were some changes that fascinated her, particularly that the Tilley lamp was no longer hanging from its hook on one of the dark brown old wooden beams running the length of the ceiling. The stain marks from the water that dripped down it in nineteen forty-seven after the big snow followed by the thaw, were still visible. The loft was full of snow that bad winter and with the thaw, it melted and dripped through the bedroom to the kitchen. The roof was fixed, but the stain marks remained as a reminder of what happened and were still pointed out to visitors on occasions. The Tilley lamps, two of them, originally one for inside and one for outside, had been put away until later in the year when they would be needed to give light in the outside buildings. A gas light replaced the kitchen Tilley lamp and was supplied with gas from the large cylinder standing in the corner of the farmhouse kitchen. Two small chains also hung from the ceiling which, in effect, were the off and on switches for the gas light. Although there was a rather loud hissing noise when lit, it was much more convenient than the Tilley lamp and threw out a brighter glow across the kitchen. The occupants of Bankside still carried candles to see their way to bed, but this was a big improvement downstairs.

Another improvement was the piped water laid on.
'No more worries about the well drying up in the back field and the tap running at a trickle,' thought Emma, 'and dad having to fill empty milk churns with water from the beck like he did one summer.' The cold-water tap, in the back kitchen, that had been their only access to water from the well, now gave out a permanent supply of water. 'Something I take for granted at the convent,' mused Emma, 'but life is so different here.' She realised that the never-ending supply was still a novelty to the family as they were forever referring to the marvel of having water even in the driest spells of summer.

Life each day, ticked over at the steady slow continuous pace of country ways. Morning and evening, milking the cows took quite a chunk out of the day. Emma was not at all interested in this work, at which Martha was very accomplished having had lots of practise. Emma helped Mary inside with the clothes to be washed and hung out in the orchard to dry and washing the cement floor, plus baking. Baking day was quite a novelty with Jacob constantly asking for tastes of the sponge mixtures and Amy insisting that she could help. Emma gave Amy her own piece of pastry to roll out and assisted her in making jam tarts. The pastry was too thinly rolled, and an overuse of jam caused it to spill over the sides of the tarts.

'I can do it myself,' Amy said. 'Don't help me,' she insisted, pushing Emma away as she tried to help.

'She is quite a little madam,' thought Emma. When the tarts were cooked, Amy proudly showed them to the family. At tea-time, every member of the family was expected to eat one. Emma thought the frustrating job of over-seeing Amy was very worthwhile when she saw her face, a picture of delight, at Tom's praise of his daughter for her deliciously tasting jam tart. Helping with housework and caring for her younger brothers and sister were a large part of her school holidays. There was plenty of enjoyment though as they went on many walks and paddled in the beck at the bottom of the pasture.

'Just like old times,' thought Emma. 'I do love it here especially in the summer.' Once back home, she soon forgot about the regime of study and the disciplined life at boarding school.

Emma also loved spending time in the evenings with Martha, after milking time, when the little ones were in bed. Martha and Emma were sharing the double bed in the sitting room which was where they spent time in private conversations. Now thirteen and becoming quite a well-developed girl for her age, Martha was showing interest in boys. Emma listened as her sister recounted some of her brief encounters with lads.

'Do you really want to know?' she asked Emma.

'Go on, tell me,' Emma replied, quite happy to listen to anything Martha was eager to share and realising that her sister wanted to tell her tale.

'I went with dad one day over to Uncle Jack's. They haven't told me yet anything much about him, but you know, Emma, he looks a bit like our dad. I think possibly he is related.

Maybe he will tell us when we're older as dad never talks about him, but they get on fine.'

'Funny, you should say that, Martha. When you wrote about dad suggesting we can call him *Uncle*, it set me thinking about how his looks and I thought maybe he's a long-lost relative.'

'Anyway,' continued Martha, wanting to relate her story, 'there was a young lad in Uncle Jack's kitchen. He looked interesting. He was tallish with long black hair and wearing overalls, but I don't know who he was and he quickly disappeared outside when we turned up. I'll tell you more if I see him again. I thought he was good looking. Maybe he just helps occasionally, but if he's local, he might come to the dances at Windrush. Dad took me once, you know. It's quite weird. All the lads sit down one side of the village hall and the girls are on the opposite side. The lads come over to ask a girl to dance with them. Dad danced with me a couple of times and I'm beginning to get the hang of it.' She smiled at Emma, expecting a response of some kind.

'I might try and learn at school as they have an old record player and sometimes at recreation, after night prayers, one of the boarders puts a record on and a few of them get up and dance together in twos. I could try,' Emma offered, 'couldn't I. Then I'll be able to go with you.'

'That sounds a good idea,' replied Martha. 'We could dance sometimes together, as I've seen other girls do that, dance together, that is, if dad lets you go. You might have to wait until you're thirteen though, like I had to.'

'There was another time I must tell you about,' Martha continued, 'when dad took me on the tractor one Saturday to that farm not far from here on the other side of the valley but further over. High Acres, I think it's called. Dad was having a long talk with the farmer and I wandered off around the buildings, just nosing about. A teenage lad, two or three years older than us probably, came face to face with me. He was quite tall with light brown wavy hair and a big smile on his face as he approached me. I kind of sidled past him but as I was passing, he patted me gently on my head and his smile widened. Then he winked at me. I remember blushing as I kept going to the end of the building before glancing back just in time to see him looking over his shoulder at me.

I had this real pleasant feeling inside me, a kind of happy, excited feeling. A bit strange really. I wonder who he was. I've been once before to that farm but didn't see him that time.'

'What did you do then?' queried Emma, trying to show interest in Martha's tale. Boys, to her, were just like her older brother, Tim, good for a joke or a laugh. She sensed that Martha's interest in them was a little different to hers.

'I wandered around the buildings hoping to catch sight of him again and found myself feeling quite disappointed when I heard dad shouting. I didn't see him as I walked back to the tractor and Dad was ready to go home. He'd finished sorting out whatever he'd gone for. Maybe he will take me next time he goes if it's when I'm off school on a Saturday and I might be able to find out about that lad. If I go during term time, I'll write and tell you. It depends if mam lets me go with dad, 'cos when you're not here, I usually help her more, instead of being outside. I like chatting to the lads when I bump into them at church or at the shop in Windrush. They seem to like me too. It's fun. Don't tell mam and dad about all this as we don't want grown-ups to think we're talking about lads, do we. They might think we're too young. I never mention it to dad.'

'Don't worry. I won't say anything. I'm glad you tell me though. Our secret. Let me know if you hear any more about Uncle Jack, though, won't you. We'd better go to sleep now.'

No sooner had Emma arrived home than it seemed the holiday was over. Mary was ironing her clothes and packing for her.

'I'll do that,' offered Emma. 'They'll only get creased in the case, anyway. Don't be bothering too much with ironing them.' Mary smiled.

'I'm going to miss you, but it will be easier for you settling in this time. No longer a new girl, now.' Emma hoped so.

'Anything will be better than last year,' she thought, pensively.

Edna Hunneysett

Autumn to Summer 1953

Emma struggled again to leave her family when the day
arrived to return to boarding school. Tom was taking time out
to give her a ride on the tractor over the moor to the bus stop
to catch the bus to Scarborough.

'Don't cry in front of your mam when we leave,' he
whispered to her, as he picked up her case to take it out to
the tractor. It only upsets her and then, the little ones get
upset as well.' Emma hugged her mam and each of her
siblings.

'I'll miss you all so much, especially you, little fellow,' she
said to Jacob, hugging him tightly. She swallowed hard and
fought back her tears until the tractor turned the corner at
the bottom of the road field, as they called it, because the
track went up the side of this field. Then her tears flowed.
Tom put his arm around his daughter whilst holding the
steering wheel with the other one.

'Come on, lass. No sooner you'll be there than it'll be half-
term and you'll be home again,' he said, trying to comfort
her. 'Here, light me one of these, will you,' he asked, passing
her a packet of woodbines and a box of matches. The girls
thought they were growing up when Tom let them light a
cigarette for him. She dried her tears and lighting the
woodbine, passed it to her dad. After parking his tractor on
the edge of the moor, Tom took Emma's case and they
crossed over the road together but struggled to find words
while they waited.

Soon Emma spied the red bus in the distance. She turned to
Tom and he gave her a hug, reducing her to tears again.
'Well, I won't have to do that if that's the effect I have on
you,' he said, jokingly. She smiled and wiped her tears as
the bus pulled up. She climbed the steps and took her case
from Tom.

'Keep smiling, lass,' he stated. Emma couldn't speak as she
watched her dad make his way back across the road to the
tractor. With a lingering look, she waved one last time as he
slowly disappeared from her sight.

Emma turned and walked up the aisle to a chorus of shouts
from girls at the back of the bus.

'Up here.'
'Come on. There's a spare seat here.' Emma approached
the back seat where the girls were sitting. Heaving her case
along, she managed to fit it in the gangway but leaving
enough room for other passengers to squeeze past it, before
taking the empty space next to Maria.
'Did you have a good holiday?' Maria asked. She was trying
to be cheerful, but looking a little weepy herself, still feeling
the pull of saying goodbye to her bunch of siblings.'
'Yes, thanks. Nothing spectacular but it was good to be at
home. Plenty of work and kids to mind. I'm sure you're the
same,' Emma added, looking at Maria. Her North Yorkshire
accent was coming through after spending weeks at home.
Maria smiled. Soon the girls were chatting away as the bus
stopped and started many times on the journey to
Scarborough. Eventually arriving at the bus station, they all
alighted and made their way through the streets, before,
once again, finding themselves outside the big, wooden
doors of the convent.

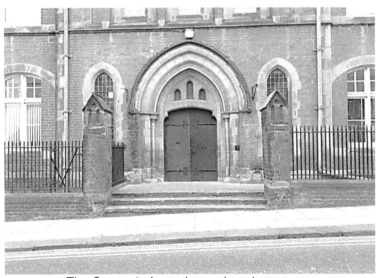

The Convent - Imposing main entrance

It was easier this term for Emma to settle down, being
familiar with the discipline and routine. As the boarders

hauled their cases up the flights of stairs, she recognised
most of the girls. She looked around, hoping to see Faith but
there was no sign of her. On reaching the dormitory,
everyone was curious to find out which cubicle they'd been
allocated. The cubicles on the garden side were the
favourite ones as only boarders who slept there, went down
that side. It was quiet and private compared with the centre
or street aisles. The occupants of the junior dormitory
walked past the street cubicles every time they went to their
dormitory. In the centre aisle, one couldn't get away with a
quiet chat because of the watchful eye of the supervising
nun sitting at her table.
'Emma, you are still in the junior dormitory,' called out
Mother Monica as Emma hovered in the doorway of the
main dormitory, waiting in the queue to read the list on the
small table. 'Some of the new boarders are already down
there. They may need a little help or advice. Just keep an
eye on them please. I will come down shortly.' Emma smiled
and nodded, but inwardly, her heart sank. She was hoping
for a cubicle and privacy, but instead, realised she'd be one
of the older ones in the junior dormitory.
'Bad luck,' whispered Audrey, who was standing behind her.
'Someone has to stay back. You shouldn't be so good,' she
added, laughingly. 'It doesn't pay. I've brought more books if
you want to borrow one.'
'Thanks, Audrey. I'll get one later. Have you seen Faith?'
'Yes, she'll be up shortly. She went into the chapel for a
quiet prayer. Her mother isn't well. She was worried about
leaving her.'

Emma sauntered around the corner to the street side and
made her way to the junior dormitory.
'Poor Faith,' she thought. 'I hope it's not serious about her
mam.' On entering the dormitory, she spotted her own name
above the first bed inside the door and put down her case on
her bed. 'Handy, when I want to get up for early Mass.
That's something, at least,' she thought. She glanced around
and immediately felt sorry for these newcomers as they
gazed at her with worried faces. 'I remember what I felt like
when I first came, the trauma of it all,' she was thinking.
'They seem so young.' One youngster was quietly crying,
sitting on her bed. Another girl seemed to be on the verge of

tears. They looked lost. Emma noticed Susanna's name above a bed. 'So, she's still in here,' she thought. Other names she recognised but those boarders weren't around. 'Possibly already in the boarders' room,' she mused, noticing that their beds were made.

'Hello. I'm Emma,' she announced. 'I was in here last year and I know the ropes. If you don't know where to put stuff or where to go, feel free to ask me. You'll notice that there are only five wash basins but ten beds. So, it's two to a basin. You'll have to take turns and don't get dressed in a morning until you've had a wash.' She looked at their worried faces. 'I remember feeling lost and lonely last year when I first arrived, but it's not so bad,' she continued. 'You'll soon feel more at home.' Emma stopped talking. 'Wrong choice of word,' she thought, as the girl on the far bed started crying again. She went over to her. 'Come on. Cheer up. It's quite bearable, this place, really. You can share a basin with me if you like, seeing as we all have to double up.' The tears subsided. 'There's one other thing,' added Emma, as she looked up at the others. 'Normally it is silence in here but today we can talk quietly whilst we sort things out.' Then she wandered back to her own bed and began to unpack.

Coming back after summer, Emma found, was quite interesting, because although knowing the routine, it was finding out the nitty-gritty of placements at table, or bath and hair wash times. Going into the boarders' room, she noticed a group of girls scanning the lists to see whether they were on early bath time or the later time. If on the earlier slot, it meant one missed the daily walk which was a bonus to some girls especially the older ones who felt it a little demeaning to have to walk in a crocodile with a nun in supervision. Piano practise lists were pinned to the notice board giving times, days and in which room one practised. Some pianos were in much better condition than others. Hence the interest in the allocation of rooms. Downstairs in the refectory were more lists showing at which table one sat for meals. Some girls were delighted and others disappointed as it wasn't just a question of whether one liked the girls, but some brought more extras than others and there were one or two fortunate enough to receive regular food parcels giving more enjoyment to the meals.

Emma finally caught up with Faith at evening recreation.
'I'm sorry to hear about your mam not being well. Audrey told me. I guess your holiday hasn't been up to much.' She hesitated, not knowing what else to say.

'Mam hasn't been very well all summer. Rose tried to get her to go to the doctors, but she wouldn't go. I don't know what's wrong with her.' At this point, the conversation ceased as the nun was clapping her hands for silence and the girls lined up to go to the dormitories. Faith was now in a cubicle on the garden side.

'Lucky you,' said Emma, when Faith told her. 'Maybe I'll get one next year.'

`Here she is,' called out Peg, next morning, when Emma walked into her form room, almost at the end of the queue.
'How was it on the farm for weeks, then?' Peg was interested in Emma's home life, so different from her own. Most of the girls were standing around chatting. A different set of girls this year as some were in the other Form III and a few from there were joining this one. Faith was among those who'd been transferred and Rita, another boarder, was one of the intakes.

'Hello, Emma.' Rita smiled, her long fringe almost covering her dark eyebrows with her cropped black hair framing her round chubby face. She wasn't very tall either. Emma was already two inches taller. She didn't know Rita very well, even though she was a boarder and they both started the same year. She was a quiet girl who kept to herself quite a lot.

'So, you're with us, this year. That's nice,' responded Emma, graciously. She wondered why pupils were moved around but she guessed there must be good reasons. Emma smiled at Peg to acknowledge her question and was just about to reply when the form teacher re-appeared. A different one this school year as Mother Catherine stayed in her own form room with a new intake of pupils.

The girls quickly went to their desks and waited in silence. The teacher was Miss Markey, their maths teacher from last year. She was short and plump with wispy, grey hair and wearing spectacles.

'Good morning, girls. The first term of a new school year. Let's hope it is a good one for you all. Leave your report books on my desk after this lesson. Can someone hand out these exercise books, please.' Emma was happy. She liked Maths. She also remembered from what some of the boarders said last year that Rita was also clever at this subject. Rita was sitting in the next desk to Emma, across the gangway.

'We'll be able to discuss maths problems together,' she thought. This pleased her.

Although Emma enjoyed the weekend walks, she found the daily weekday walk a bit tedious. When she discovered that a handful of boarders were in the school choir and because of this, missed a weekly walk, she decided to join them. 'I think it's a good idea,' she explained to Faith, one evening, 'because the weekly choir practise is straight after school. I need permission to miss the walk but that's okay as the others have permission. I'll be able to miss it once a week. Apparently, by the time choir practise is over and if the rest of the boarders aren't back, I'll be able to wander up to the boarders' room and have a chat with any girls around, or just read, with no-one there supervising.' Emma was considering this later when lying in bed. 'It'll be a sense of freedom for a short while,' she thought. 'A bit like getting up for Mass when the others don't.'

'That's a lovely dress, Emma,' called out one of the girls coming into the boarders' room the following Saturday morning. 'I thought it was Audrey on the stairs in front of me until you turned around, as she has one similar, hasn't she,' she stated.

'I know what you're thinking,' mused Emma. 'You think my parents can't afford a dress like this and you're right. They can't.' But she didn't voice these thoughts. She smiled in acknowledgement and went to sit down. At home, the children changed from their good clothes into ones which were often hand-me-downs or clothes they'd been given from relatives. Here, at boarding school, the girls also changed into their own clothes in the evenings and wore them at weekends. Emma was conscious of her very limited wardrobe, alternating between one of two new jumpers with a skirt or three cotton dresses in the warmer weather. Audrey sometimes wore a dress that was bright and shiny with many different colours and made of taffeta and with double turn-up cuffs. It made swishing noises as Audrey moved about. Emma thought the dress was beautiful.

It was when the parcel arrived in the summer holidays from Mary's friend who lived away and was married to a headmaster, that she was over the moon to find amongst the second-hand but nearly new selection of clothes, a dress like Audrey's. 'It's a bit tight on me,' she'd stated to her mother whilst doing a little swirl in the farmhouse kitchen, 'but I can still wear it.' She'd felt self-conscious, but proud, when walking into the boarders' room until the comment was made. Sitting quietly doing her homework, she was wondering if she shouldn't have worn it, if it stands out that much. 'Maybe they guess it's second-hand,' she thought, feeling embarrassed. 'I don't think I'll wear it again and I'll tell mam that it was a bit too tight after all.' Emma felt decidedly glum.

The weeks ticked by. Faith was eager to get home for half-term to see her mother. Although she was receiving a weekly letter from her, Faith sensed that things weren't right with her mam. She was also struggling with another problem and didn't know quite what to do about it. She was too embarrassed to discuss it with anyone, but her uniform dress was becoming tighter across her chest and whilst Faith was feeling uncomfortable with it, she didn't like to ask her mam for money for a larger size, especially as her mam was unwell. Eventually, towards the end of breakfast one morning, the problem was resolved when Mother Teresa tapped her on the shoulder.

'Come with me.' Faith, looking worried, folded her serviette and put it in the ring before leaving the table. She followed the nun along the corridor and up the stairs. They stopped outside the large wardrobe at the end of the second corridor. 'I think you'll be better in a blouse and skirt, as you're growing so quickly. Take these,' she said, handing Faith the school uniform clothes. 'They look about your size. Go and change into them and leave your dress on your bed. I'll collect it.' Faith thanked her and feeling very relieved, went straight to the dormitory, whilst wondering how she was going to explain this to Emma. She felt awkward telling anyone.

'Your uniform looks great,' Emma whispered, a little later, as they stood together in the hall for assembly. 'Did Mother Teresa sort you out?' Faith looked surprise at this question but nodded, uncomfortably.

'How did you guess?'

'She did that for me the very first morning, as my dress was faded and horrible. She was very kind. Don't worry about me knowing. I won't tell anyone,' reassured Emma. 'I told no-one about me.' Faith smiled, almost in tears with relief. 'Thanks,' was all she could say.

Unlike her first few months at school, Emma no longer worried about conversation with the day girls. She knew that she spoke more clearly and correctly, but there were times when she felt ignorant on topics that came up. More worryingly was when, on occasions, her concentration slipped and her accent became more pronounced, as happened on the last Sunday evening before half-term. Supper time was brought forward and this was the sign that something was going to happen. They were to have a treat. The nuns had obtained a projection and screen and there was great excitement among the boarders as word spread around that they were going to have a film show. All the tables in the boarders' room were pushed to one side and the chairs placed in rows so that everyone could sit together. Then all the nuns trooped in and took up places behind the girls. Even Mother Margaret came along. The lights went out and the film started rolling.

The projector made a whirring sound as it threw the pictures onto the screen at the other end of the boarders' room. Emma was fascinated even at the roar of the lion at the beginning. She became very tense, completely absorbed by the story, feeling almost a part of the actions, suffering the anxieties and enjoying the good bits almost as if she were in the film. She heard one of the older nuns tut-tutting at the kissing bits.

'So unhygienic,' she heard her comment from a few rows behind.' Emma smiled to herself.

'What a great film,' she whispered to Faith, immediately after *The End* appeared on the screen. She pronounced film as *filum*.

'It's film, not *filum*. Your pronunciation! What's it like!' Faith commented, but she was smiling so as not to upset her friend. Once again, Emma felt embarrassed and shy, conscious of her accent and feeling different.

'Another word I must remember to pronounce correctly,' she thought. The lights went on and everyone gazed around at all the red faces, some a little tearful and others looking tired as it was past their usual bedtime and quite late for the junior dormitory boarders. Emma felt exhilarated. She was mentally adding to her list of names of film stars such as Stewart Grainger, Robert Mitchum and Gregory Peck, two or three more main actors from the film. She didn't feel any desire to swoon over them like some of the older girls but at least she felt able to converse about their good and not so good points. Emma slept well.

Whilst Emma's confidence was growing, she still had fears to overcome. One Friday afternoon towards the end of term, with a double lesson of English on the timetable, the teacher decided that the pupils would play charades but with relevance to literature.

'You will all form into groups of three please. Each group, in turn, will come to the front and act out a very short sketch from the Shakespeare play we've been studying this term. The rest of you will try and guess what is being acted. You won't have much time. Make it simple and to the point if you can. Then we'll have a vote at the end as to which group was the best.' Emma's heart sank.

'Not acting. No way,' she thought, but she didn't have a chance to not participate.

'Come and join us,' called out Mavis, a freckled-faced, chubby pupil who was good at literature and who'd teamed up with Anthea with whom she was friendly. Anthea, beside her, her fringe of straight black hair almost in her eyes, nodded.

'Come on, Emma. You'll be fine with us,' she said. Anthea was in a theatrical group and on occasions, enjoyed being part of a production at the local theatre. Looking for a third person, they both thought that because she was clever as well as being generally chatty and pleasant with everyone, she'd be fine and help them win, but Emma knew otherwise. When it came to public speaking, Emma was tongue-tied and shy. Another tall girl, Brenda, very outgoing and bursting with confidence, hand-picked two others, making what she thought was a strong group to outshine the rest. The charades began. Each group spent a short time planning their sketch before going to the front, facing their audience and presenting their charade. Whilst Mavis and Anthea acted with conviction, Emma was wooden and stilted and her words very flat. She knew she'd let them down when they came runners up to Brenda's group who were voted outstanding.

'Sorry,' Emma whispered.

'Don't worry,' Mavis replied. 'You tried.' Anthea didn't comment. She was disappointed.

Term time finally came to an end and the boarders left for home after many goodbyes.

'Enjoy as best you can, time with your mam and I'll see you next term,' were Emma's parting words to her friend, but then wondered if she'd said the right thing. A couple of weeks back, Faith had read out to Emma a few lines of her last letter from her sister Rose. It seemed to Emma that things were not sounding good regarding the health of her mam. As she was leaving, Faith gave Emma a weak smile.

It was the usual fun time at Christmas for Emma, back home with her family. She noticed that Tim was growing tall, like his dad. Life was bleak these winter months at Bankside farm and Emma didn't mind helping Mary in the house, rather than out in the freezing cold buildings, milking cows and mucking out. Midnight Mass was a highlight. Just as Mary was making the traditional Christmas eve giblet pie for tea, there was a knock at the door.

'See who that is, will you,' Mary said.

'No cheating,' Emma told Mark, as she got up from the clip mat where they'd been engrossed in a game of draughts. Mark grinned widely, his two dimples adding to his mischievous look of glee. 'I mean it,' she stated, making for the door. She went to open the coals door, named because of the great pile of coals stacked behind the stone wall around that side of the house.

As she reached forward to lift the sneck, the door opened
and Uncle Jack stepped inside, carrying a large bag.
'Father Christmas has arrived early,' he said, smiling
broadly. 'My, how you are growing. Home for Christmas, I
take it. Is your mam in?' Emma smiled and nodded. He
followed her into the kitchen. 'There's a good smell in here.
Cooking, are you, Mary?'
'Hello, Jack. It's good to see you. Yes, it's a ritual you know.
We always have giblet pie on Christmas eve. Stay and have
some. Tom will be in shortly.'
'I'd like that, Mary. I can't stay too long thought. Cows to be
seen to.' Jack was very fond of Mary. 'I'll pick up the family
for Midnight Mass, if you like. They'll get to bed a bit earlier if
I bring them home. Father Christmas coming, is he?' he
asked Amy, who was dancing around in excitement, her
dark brown eyes gleaming under her thick, lengthy fringe.
She loved Christmas.
'What's in there, Uncle Jack?' she asked, inquisitively.
'Surprises,' he answered, 'and to be opened tomorrow.' Amy
pulled a face.
'Can't we open just one?' she pleaded.
'Well, that's up to your mam.'
'Put them on the bed in the sitting room for now, Jack, will
you please. You are coming for dinner tomorrow, aren't you,'
Mary added, as he came back in, having deposited the bag.
'Aye. I wouldn't miss it for anything.'

Since his reconciliation with Tom, over a year ago, Jack
Netherfield spent time with him and his family and having
no-one at home, enjoyed their hospitality immensely. They,
in turn, enjoyed the luxury of his van on occasions. Emma
was studying Jack Netherfield, as her mam and he
conversed.
'Martha was right,' she thought. 'He does look like our dad. I
wonder what that story is.' Emma was beginning to read
some of the magazines that the older boarders lent her. She
was finding out that some families were different and
complicated with half-brothers and sisters. The short true-to-
life stories fascinated her although she felt they were
sometimes a bit far-fetched. Maybe when she was thirteen

and allowed to go to the local dance with Martha, Uncle Jack
might pick them up and then they could possibly ask him.
'Emma,' shouted Mark, snapping her out of her daydream,
'are we going to finish this game?'

Arriving back in January after the Christmas holidays, Emma
was making her way out of the dormitory to take her case to
the attic when Mother Monica stopped her in her tracks.
'Emma, I need to see you in my office please,' and looking at
her watch, added, 'in about ten minutes.'
'Yes Mother,' Emma replied dutifully, but inside she felt a
little sick. She thought Mother Monica was quite strict.
'What's this about,' she wondered. She soon found out. She
took her case to the attic and greeting some girls on route,
made her way to Mother Monica's office, knocking timidly on
the door.
'Come in,' the voice called. 'Hello, Emma. Just close the
door behind you please. Did you enjoy Christmas with your
family?'
'Very much,' Emma replied, still wondering why she'd been
call in. 'I've had a lovely holiday, thank you, Mother.'
'You are quite friendly with Faith, aren't you?' Mother Monica
questioned. Emma nodded. 'I have some sad news for you.'
It was then that Mother Monica explained that Faith's mother
died four days after Christmas day. Emma was shocked.
'Poor Faith. How awful,' she thought. 'Is she coming back?'
she ventured to ask.
'Yes, but as you can imagine, she has not had a happy
Christmas. So be aware of this when you meet up. I am sure
you will be very sympathetic towards her. Let her talk about
it, if she wishes to. She may, however, not be ready and if
that is the case, just say how sorry you are and leave it
there. She will need time, no doubt, but if you are around,
she may eventually confide in you.' Emma nodded. She was
dumfounded. 'Thank you, Emma. You may go now.'

Emma walked out of the office and almost immediately
bumped into Faith who was just coming up the stairs.
'Faith, I'm so sorry. Mother Monica has just told me. Faith's
eyes welled up.
'It's been an awful Christmas,' she began. They stepped to

one side and began talking in little whispers as other girls passed up and down the stairs. 'No-one met me at the station and I walked home feeling very alone. My mam...' She gulped and wiped her eyes. 'Sorry.' Emma put her arm around her friend, feeling so bad about how she'd spent a lovely Christmas with her family whilst Faith had been going through this.

'Don't apologise. You can talk to me about it, if you wish.' Faith shook her head.

'I will, but not just now, if you don't mind. I'm struggling just having people mention it. I need to get through these next few days. Being here will help though, to take my mind off it. I will tell you, Emma. I'm glad you're my friend.' Her eyes were filling up again. Emma gave her a quick hug.

As the days passed, Faith told Emma, little by little, of the days leading up to her mam's death. At the time it happened, Faith was too numb to take it in and although she'd spent hours by her mam's bedside until four days after Christmas, when her mam finally passed away, Faith only remembered it all as a blur in her mind. A week or so later, at recreation time, Faith voiced another concern.

'You know my sister, Rose. Well, she helped me to get through it, but she was so upset, too. She works and isn't at home much, as I've said in the past. Now my uncles don't know what to do with me and I don't know what I will do at half-term.' Emma gave this some thought and in a letter home, asked if she might bring Faith back with her on one of the holidays. Mary wasn't sure about having a school friend of Emma's come to spend time at Bankside, having lived in a town before marrying Tom and knowing that it was a lot different from their existence on this isolated farm. She felt uncertain about replying to the request, before having a chat with her daughter. Mary knew that some would find conditions difficult at Bankside, if they were used to a more civilised life in a town. Faith would have to share a bed too, she thought. Mary told Emma in her letter that they'd discuss the matter at half-term.

It was a couple of weeks into the term, when the humiliating game of charades, played in the English lesson, came back to haunt Emma. Anthea stood up one morning in class just as the break bell went and asked to speak to everyone for a moment.

'As some of you know,' she began, tucking her straight hair behind her ear, 'I'm very interested in drama and attend a local theatrical group. I've been in a couple of productions. Some of you go to ballet lessons and I understand that we have a couple of talented singers amongst us. Mavis and I are thinking of putting on a play at the end of this term. We'll have to ask permission, but before that, we'd like to know if any of you are interested in taking part.' Mavis, who was standing at the far side of the form room, joined in.

'It will be great fun. We could rehearse at lunch time or after school and in small groups at first before we put the whole thing together. If you would like to be part of the planning or have ideas that you'd like to share, stay behind now and we'll have a ten-minute discussion, or if you are interested in taking part when it gets underway, just leave your name with one of us. Thanks.' For a moment, there was silence as this information was digested. A few of the pupils then made for the door, Emma included. This wasn't her scene at all and although, over the following weeks to half-term, Emma was constantly being informed of the progress of the production as more form pupils joined in, she wasn't interested in participating.

'Did you ask?' enquired Faith, on their return after the four-day break. 'Emma looked downcast knowing she would be disappointing her friend.

'Mam said that they thought it would be best to come in summer as Easter holidays are short and the weather is better in summer. Sorry.'

'It's all right. It will be something to look forward to. Thanks for asking.' With that, the topic was closed for the time being.

As the term progressed, the girls were becoming more animated about their production. They welcomed the enthusiasm and encouragement from their English teacher who was ready to give advice when asked. Eventually, Mavis, who was mostly in charge of the organising, asked everyone including Emma, to meet after dinner, one Friday afternoon.

'Thank you all for coming,' Anthea announced, pushing her

black fringe to one side. 'Mavis has asked me to explain. We have had great interest in our production and almost all of you are now involved. Because of this, we feel that we'd like to give everyone a small part.' At this point, Mavis looked at Emma. 'Emma,' Anthea said, 'I know you are not bothered about being in it, but we don't want to leave anyone out. We have given you a very small part. You too, Laura, as you are the other one not taking part, but if you will come along as well, that will be everyone. How do you feel about that, both of you?' Emma turned around to glance at Laura, tall and broad with light brown, wavy hair, who was looking back at her, questioningly. She was a quiet, good-natured girl, who mostly kept to herself. She'd spoken to Emma a few times and offered her sweets on occasions. She lived outside Scarborough in a small village and when in their form room, always sat at the very back. 'If you two will come to the next rehearsal,' continued Anthea, 'we will explain, but it is very simple. You have little to say and only one brief walk across the stage. What do you think?' The two girls exchanged further glances, before both nodding.

The next day after dinner, Emma went to the main hall to find all the girls chatting and buzzing around whilst Brenda, in her usual very confident and rather bossy manner, was directing some of them into their places on the stage.
'I've got this grand title of producer,' she said, laughingly, as the two girls approached, 'ably assisted by Anthea of course, with Mavis being overall director. This is what we'd like you to do. You walk onto the stage, when it's your turn in the scene, and you just must act like two elderly ladies who are going shopping and are putting the world to rights as you go. Just make anything up as it will only last a couple of minutes. There are plenty of clothes in the store cupboard for you to choose an outfit from. Does that sound okay?' Laura and Emma smiled.
'Not so bad, after all,' Emma decided, quite relieved. She managed her small part on the opening night, although someone commented that they couldn't hear what Laura and she were saying to each other. 'You weren't meant to. We were just two elderly ladies having a chat whilst walking to the shops,' Emma explained, smiling to herself. Another barrier she'd overcome. The play was a success and

performed in the hall in front of many pupils with their teachers just before the end of term.

Summer term brought extra joy for Emma. Firstly, there was tennis which she was learning to play and could practise at recreation in the evenings as the boarders spent this time outside on the courts in the convent grounds. There were benches where the girls chatted together, or one could curl up in a corner of one for a quiet read. Some girls walked around the perimeter of the grounds for exercise. The light nights meant that she could read in bed too, long after the time that lights were normally switched off. Having discovered the joys of the swimming pool, Emma was delighted when Faith told her about a group of boarders who were planning to go swimming once a week after school hours and was asked if she'd like to join them. As well as Faith, there was Audrey along with two or three older boarders. These girls, having asked permission, missed the walk by going to the refectory for an early tea of bread and jam before wandering through the streets of Scarborough to the swimming baths. Emma loved this weekly trip to the pool where, although still not having managed to swim a width, loved being able to splash around, practise her strokes and have slides down the chute. The school choir practises ceased at Easter, but now, missing the walk to go swimming once a week compensated. The girls loved an hour away from the orderly and disciplined regime of life in boarding school with its silences and restrictions.

'What do you think about the planned pilgrimage to Walsingham?' Faith asked, when she met up with Emma at break time, one Monday. It had been announced at the morning assembly by Mother Monica that a school pilgrimage was being organised to visit The Shrine of Our Lady of Walsingham in Norfolk, at the invitation of Mother Superior. A special attraction was a large, coloured-glass window, known as The East Window, which had recently been installed above the altar in the Slipper Chapel. The installation of this window was to commemorate the formal definition of the Dogma of The Assumption of Our Lady, declared by the Pope in 1950.
'I've never been anywhere like that. Let's put our names

down,' replied Emma. 'I'd love a trip out even though Mother Monica said it was a long journey to go there and back in a day, but that won't matter to us.'

It was a long day, but Emma and Faith, sitting together on the coach, thoroughly enjoyed it. They each brought with them their packed lunches. Mother Monica had let those boarders who were going, take their purses from her office, although both girls had little spare money. Dismounting from the coaches, the party sauntered through the village before walking the mile up a lane to the shrine. They ate lunch in the open air followed by Mass outside. Sitting outside on wooden benches in the sunshine was very different to a Mass in church or chapel, and Emma enjoyed the experience, especially the singing. The girls wandered around freely afterwards and Emma was amazed at the fourteen huge, oak crosses erected at intervals outside, denoting The Way of the Cross, so unlike the small pictures inside the convent chapel. As well as viewing the beautiful large East Window, depicting in glowing colours the glorious Assumption of Our Lady, they visited the gift shop where there was a large selection of rosary beads, prayer cards, missals and statues.

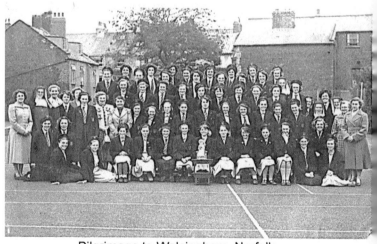

Pilgrimage to Walsingham, Norfolk

'I think I'll buy a prayer card,' whispered Faith. From the large selection, they each chose one and paid at the counter before re-entering the chapel to kneel together for private prayer. On leaving the chapel, they went outside to find that their coach had arrived. It was time to leave.

When arriving back at the convent, everyone congregated on the tennis courts in the convent grounds for a group photo. The youngest pilgrim, in the centre of the front row, was holding a statue of Our Lady of Walsingham, that was to be placed in the convent chapel.
'It's been a great day,' Emma whispered to Faith, on their way to the dormitories. 'Sleep well,' she added, before turning left to go to the junior dormitory.

The weeks seemed to pass quickly. The end of term was approaching.
'Are you sure, it's all right for me to come?' questioned Faith, yet again. Emma, having repeated her request when she was at home at Easter about Faith coming and wanting reassurance that her friend could indeed spend time on the farm in the summer holidays, was happy that Tom and Mary agreed.
'I told you that I talked with mam and dad at Easter about you coming in summer. They don't mind provided I explain honestly what it's like on our farm. There is no bathroom or anything, you know that, and you will have to sleep with me. But if you're okay with that, then it's fine.'
'I really want to come, Emma. It's so miserable at home. Rose is hardly there. I think she stays at her boyfriend's house and my uncles are out a lot. I would love to come.'
'Well, that's settled then. I'll tell mam next time I write. Wait till you meet Jacob and Amy. It'll be fun.'

Faith was firstly introduced to Emma's dad when Tom picked them up and gave them a lift home from the bus stop, on his tractor. Emma was feeling nervous about bringing Faith to her home. She explained again about having no bathroom and that the outside toilet consisted of a bucket under a wooden seat with no flush.
'You'll be sleeping with me downstairs in a double bed, if that's okay,' she added, forgetting that she'd already

mentioned this to Faith. Whatever she told her, it didn't seem to matter to Faith or diminish her joy at the thought of spending time on the farm. After arriving at Bankside with Emma, she took everything in her stride. If it was an eye-opener for her, she didn't show it. Nothing seemed to phase her. She radiated happiness and was willing to help, wherever needed. She took Amy and little Jacob for walks, played draughts with Mark and learnt how to play cards, with Tom teaching her, in the evenings. Tom cracked jokes with her, whilst the younger children commandeered her attention.

On Sunday morning, as usual, Tom took some of the family including Faith, to the second Mass of the morning, on the tractor, Mark and Tim having been to the earlier Mass. Mary sat on the double seat with Jacob on her knee, leaving the two friends and little Amy to sit in the wooden link-box attached to the back of the tractor. Never having ridden on a tractor until coming to Bankside, Faith found it very exciting. Like everything else that happened, she accepted and joyously took on board this latest event. She thought the icing on the cake was riding to church on the tractor.
'It's great doing this,' she commented, as the tractor chugged its way down the tarmac road. Emma smiled, relieved that her friend was enjoying the experience on the farm. Emma loved her family but was concerned about the living conditions when bringing her friend to such a lifestyle as theirs, at Bankside. She now wondered if maybe Faith's home was not much different.
'It must be hard living with bachelor uncles and with no-one else to see to the cooking and cleaning,' she thought, 'especially with her sister, Rose, often staying at her boyfriend's. I doubt she'll ever invite me to her home. Not that it matters. It's probably more fun here for Faith.'

The holiday for Faith wasn't to last, as a week into it, a letter addressed to Emma, arrived from The Farmers Weekly office. The postman delivered the letter just as the family were finishing a late dinner. Emma opened it, with trepidation, as everyone watched.
'Well?' questioned Mary. 'What does it say?' Emma's dark eyes were shining.

'I've won. I'm one of the winners. I'm going on a thirteen-day trip.' She passed the letter to her mother to read. This real holiday, as she began calling it, was because Emma was one of a group of outright winners from the annual competition run monthly by The Farmers Weekly magazine. Even during the school term, Emma faithfully kept up to date with her monthly competition entries which covered various topics of writing accompanied by a drawing to illustrate the story. Mary had written to Mother Monica about the competition at the beginning of the school year for permission for Emma to send the first entry by the end of September. The headmistress replied that she was happy for Emma to submit monthly entries provided it did not interfere with her studies. Mary was pleased as she encouraged her children to participate in these competitions and they'd already won a few prizes over the years when entering in the younger age group. At the end of each month leading up to the end of June, prizes were given to the first, second and third winners plus a few consolation prizes for the runners-up. Emma delighted in seeing her name in print and she'd received books as prizes when she came in the monthly top three. The books weren't Enid Blyton's or girlie books but were more educational and she didn't always find them interesting but one or two of them she'd enjoyed reading, such as *Tarka the Otter* and *Over the hills with Nomad*.

The previous year, Martha was one of the youngest winners in the older section of the competition. She'd made the long journey to an Educational College near Shrewsbury. The students had dispersed for the summer, making it an ideal place for the prize winners and staff of The Farmers Weekly. Emma remembered how excited Martha was before she went and how she'd talked about this wonderful experience for the rest of the summer holidays. She'd described visiting a brewery and a tannery. They'd been to farms looking at different up-to-date machinery and Martha was so impressed seeing a modern milking parlour. Sometimes there was afternoon tea of sandwiches, cakes and buttered scones in the farmhouse kitchen, after the group finished inspecting the farm.
'And now it's my turn,' Emma thought, feeling excited.

'You can stay a few more days,' stated Mary, turning to Faith. 'Then we will have to make preparation for Emma's trip. You can come again to stay. It's been lovely having you and you've been a good help with the younger children.' Faith smiled, trying to hide her disappointment at having to leave sooner than expected. She was hoping that she might be able to stay the whole of the holidays.

'You're so lucky, Emma, having a family like this,' she said, on the morning she was leaving to go home. 'Thanks for inviting me.'

'I'll ask mam about Christmas, if you like. Maybe we'll get to a dance together. They're only once a month at Windrush. So, you'll miss the next one.' Faith said she'd think about it as her sister, Rose, might want her at home for Christmas but that she'd love to come again, maybe on one of the other school holidays. The invitation was left open.

As the date of Emma's trip approached, she was becoming more and more restless. She found herself distracted whilst baking for her mam as she was preoccupied at the thought of another holiday within these summer holidays and was very much looking forward to it. She'd been counting the days and tomorrow was the big day when it would all happen. During the night, Emma tossed and turned in her sleep subconsciously knowing she was to be up early tomorrow.

'Emma, can't you keep still,' mumbled Martha, at being disturbed by Emma's shuffling as she turned over and over. 'Sorry,' whispered Emma.

Mary and Tom arranged for Emma to meet up with another of the finalists, a young lady who lived outside Harrogate on a turkey farm. Tom discussed this with Jack one Sunday after church, when having a pint in the Hunters Lodge, their local at Windrush and Jack kindly offered his van for Tom to take Emma on part of the journey. The plan was that Jean's mam would meet them halfway and take Emma back to her place to stay overnight. The next day, Jean's dad was taking the two girls by car to the railway station to take a train to Shrewsbury. The girls were to be met by two representatives from The Farmers Weekly, Dot and Joan, who were meeting trains from various parts of the country and escorting the youngsters to the hotel to settle them in. There, they would meet with the winners of the competition plus other staff who would chaperone and guide them throughout the holiday.

'They suggest a list of suitable clothing for you, Emma,' stated her mother, one afternoon, on reading a further letter about the trip, delivered by the postman earlier. 'You will have to make do with what you've got, though,' she added.
'I'm sure I'll be all right. I've become more used to having less than some. It doesn't bother me much now.'
'I know what we could do, Emma. You could have a home perm,' enthused Mary, now that you're starting to grow up. Mary regularly gave herself a perm assisted by Martha who knew how to put the rollers in where it was more difficult for her mother to reach around the back of her head.
'Can I have mine done too?' questioned Martha.
'I didn't know that you were interested in having one, but of course you can, if you want to,' replied Mary, aware that her eldest daughter was developing into a young woman more quickly than some thirteen-year-old girls. 'I have a couple of kits in as I make sure I don't run out in winter. We'll have a perming day this week.' She'd noticed that Martha was paying quite a lot of attention to her appearance and her clothes, these days. She'd seen her glancing over at the boys in church and loitering after Mass to chat to them, obviously enjoying their company. 'It will be lipstick next, I suppose,' thought Mary. 'How quickly they grow up.'

Perming day arrived.
'I'll do Emma's first, Martha. You mind Jacob and Amy for me. Then Emma can swop with you when I've finished hers,' said Mary, bringing the perming kit box from the cupboard. Emma washed her hair over the bowl in the kitchen and gave it a towel rub. Mary clipped Emma's straight black hair to a suitable length, the small cuttings free-falling onto the cement floor. 'We'll sweep them up at the end,' Mary said. 'Just don't let the little ones near, Martha. You might like to take them outside for a play as it's lovely and sunny today.' Martha disappeared with Jacob and Amy and the house was much quieter. Mary placed on the table all the contents of the perming kit alongside a box of rollers kept solely for this purpose and poured half of the perming solution into a small

bowl. Then taking a few strands of Emma's hair at a time, she gently combed them before pulling them gently through the piece of cotton wool that she'd dipped into the bowl, carefully making sure that the strands were all well dampened. Following this, she took one of the small pieces of thin paper from the pack supplied in the kit and wrapping it round the wet hair strands, slid the paper to overlap the hair ends before rolling the now covered hair onto a curler. Slowly she worked until there was a row of curlers all the way from Emma's brow to the nape of her neck. Mary patiently continued by evenly forming rows of tightly wound curlers down both sides of her head. 'Now I have to use the rest of the solution by soaking the cotton wool and squeezing each curler to make sure all the curlers are well moistened,' she explained. 'Then we wait awhile before we put on the neutraliser. We'll have time for a cup of tea, I think.'

Emma got up and went to look at herself in the small slightly cracked mirror, hanging by a piece of string fastened to a nail on the wall. It was the mirror Tom used when having a shave. She smiled at herself on seeing her head covered in bright blue and red curlers. The smell of the perming solution was almost offensive and reeked around the farmhouse kitchen. At that moment, the little ones came running through the door, trying to beat Martha into the house.
'Ugh! What's that horrible smell?' asked Amy, curling the nostrils of her neat, little, snub nose. Mark followed behind, having joined them on their walk.
'It stinks,' he said.
'It's just Emma's perm. If you leave the doors open, the smell will soon disappear,' suggested Mary, pouring herself and Emma a cup of tea. 'There's more in the pot if you want one, Martha.' Tom and Tim called in for an early sandwich lunch whilst Mary was having her cup of tea.
'We'll be out in the buildings putting in water bowls ready for when we get drinking water laid on, for the cattle,' he told Mary, as they were leaving. 'Don't expect us in too early as I want to get the job finished today, if we can.' They were glad to be out of the kitchen. 'It's a much healthier smell outside in the buildings, than in there,' Tom said wryly to Tim, when out of earshot. His son grinned.

'It's time for rinsing and neutralizing, Emma,' stated her mother, checking the instructions supplied with the kit and looking at the clock. 'We will soon be finished.' She carefully poured warm water over Emma's head making sure each roller was properly rinsed. Then a squeeze of each rolled curler with a towel to take up the excess water before applying the neutralizer. A further wait and more rinsing before she finally unwound, one by one, each of the curlers, dropping them into a bowl to be washed, in readiness for Martha's perm. The younger children watched, fascinated as their mother took the curlers out, revealing tight little black curls covering Emma's head. Then Mary gently combed out the curls to leave a mass of tiny waves. 'What do you think?' she asked Emma, holding the mirror in front of her.

'Oh, my,' was all Emma could say. She found the effect startling. 'I look older,' she thought.

'Stand up,' said Mary, 'and let me have a good look.' She immediately saw that her little girl was growing up. Emma was quite tall for her age and slim too. With her short, straight hair normally clipped back, but now transformed into a mass of modern curls, it was as if she had added years to her age. 'You look lovely,' Mary said to her daughter. 'You really suit it.' Emma smiled.

'You are so pretty,' voiced Amy, in admiration.

'Thanks, Amy. You're pretty, too, you know.'

'Now, we'll have a bite to eat and then I'll do yours, Martha,' said Mary. 'Won't Tim and dad be surprised when they come in.'

A few hours later, Martha and Emma were standing staring at each other and then giggling and exclaiming. From being two young girls with straight, short hair each wearing a hairclip to hold it back from their eyes, they'd been changed into two young ladies with modern hair styles.

'I wonder what dad will say,' voiced Martha.

'Let's go and show him,' responded Emma. 'Come on. Let's go and find him.'

'Not before you've swept up the hair cuttings up, please,' stated Mary, sitting down and having a woodbine after her busy day. 'Don't be long out there either as I need a hand with the tea.' The girls quickly got the shovel and brush and swept up the hair scattered on the cement floor and tipped it onto the fire where it sizzled and burnt. The girls tore out of the house and ran down the cobbles to the cowshed, charging in and coming to a stop as Tom and Tim were just finishing the last water bowl.

'Look at us,' they chorused. Tom stopped for a moment. He wasn't too interested in all this perming lark. He thought his lasses were fine with straight hair. He kept it cut short and tidy with a regular cut and it cost nothing. Perms meant money.
'Aye, you look okay,' was his comment. Tim laughed.
'You look daft, I think,' he said. The girls, slightly subdued, but only slightly, walked back to the farmhouse.
'I think we look lovely, Martha,' Emma said, running her fingers through her curls. 'Don't you, Martha?' Martha nodded enthusiastically whilst busily thinking about what the boys might say. 'Just wait until I'm back at school,' Emma thought, wondering what her peer group might say. She was dying to show Faith.

A Real Holiday

A few days later, Emma was on her way down the country seated in the back of what she thought was a rather posh car. She was sitting behind Jean who was in the passenger seat next to her father and they were talking quietly. Emma was looking at Jean's mouse-coloured hair.
'She's not as pretty as Martha,' she thought. She'd found Jean to be a very quiet young lady over dinner the previous evening and it was Jean's mother who kept the conversation going. 'Perhaps she is shy, like me before I went to boarding school,' Emma mused, realising how her confidence was growing since being away from home. Jean's parents owned and worked a large turkey farm. Emma was amazed when shown the turkeys. There seemed to be hundreds and they were noisy. She'd never seen real turkeys before. Jean's mother explained to Emma the difficulties of rearing turkeys and the excess workload near Christmas to meet the deadlines for the buyers.

Jean was an only child and seemed a little ill at ease with Emma.
'I suppose I'm a bit boisterous for her. I probably talk too much as well,' Emma decided, after chatting to Jean about her brothers and sisters and boarding school, as the train made its way across the countryside. Jean wasn't saying much at all. 'This is difficult but better than sitting in silence,' thought Emma. 'I hope we're soon there.' After frequent stops to allow other passengers to get off or on, the train finally pulled into Shrewsbury station. The girls joined the other passengers struggling to collect their suitcases from among the luggage stacked up. When this trip for Emma came about, Mary decided to buy another case, having realised that the original large one she'd purchased for Emma's bedding, when Emma first went to boarding school, was too big and cumbersome and the other smaller one was too little as it was more of a weekend case. This one was an in-between size and much better for this trip and more suitable for school too, Mary thought. She felt it was money well spent especially as she'd seen the suitcase in a sale. Stepped down from the train, carrying her case, Emma was very pleased with her mam's decision.

'This one is much easier to handle than that big one,' she thought, 'and I like the dark blue colour better than brown.'

'Have you brought a copy of The Farmers Weekly?' asked Jean, brightening up a little, when once on the platform. Emma nodded, unzipping her hand luggage and taking from it the bright yellow-covered magazine. She rolled it up and holding it high whilst looking up and down the platform, began gently waving it to and fro, just like they'd been instructed to do in the letter each prize winner received. Jean was doing likewise with her own copy.
'There, look,' said Emma, excitedly. 'Two ladies over there holding copies in the air.' They waved their own as they made their way along the platform to meet up with The Farmers Weekly representatives. One was tall and elegantly dressed in a light grey trouser suit and low heel red shoes, matching her handbag slung over one shoulder. Her long blond hair was blowing a little in the summer breeze. The other, slightly less tall and a little chunky with close cropped auburn hair, wore a summer floral dress, pale blue jacket and white sandals.
'Hello,' they greeted the girls as they met together. 'You must be Emma Holmes and Jean Speight. I'm Joan,' said the taller of the two, 'and this is Dot. Congratulations on being final prize winners.' They smiled and shook hands with each of the girls, as Emma and Jean introduced themselves. 'Here, let me carry that for you,' Joan offered, taking Jean's case.

'I'll take your case for you, Emma,' offered the friendly smaller woman. 'I bet you're both hungry and a little tired. You are the last of the party to arrive, but you have come a fair distance. We'll go straight to the hotel and meet with the other winners and have an evening meal, all of us. Bob and Tony will be there and will look after you throughout the fortnight. The party are all waiting in the hotel lounge, but I suspect by the time we arrive, they'll be in the dining room. Have you been to this part of the country before, either of you?' she questioned, as they walked past a railway official and along to the taxi rank. The girls shook their heads. Emma was a little apprehensive but so glad that she'd had her hair permed. It gave her confidence to know that she looked 'bonny' as Mary said, as she knew that was a compliment.

'The Star Hotel, please,' Joan instructed the cab driver, once they'd settled inside the taxi. Emma's only knowledge of a taxi was the one at Windrush but that was just an ordinary car run by a local villager. She'd never been inside one like this, big and black with folding-up seats opposite the ones they were sitting on. The taxi driver took their luggage and placed it in the boot before getting into his seat and driving off.

Arriving at the hotel after a very short journey, the little party alighted from the taxi and collected the luggage after the driver placed it upon the kerb. Joan paid him the fare and asked for a receipt whilst the girls followed Dot. They were both now feeling slightly anxious and remained silent. Dot walked into the small hotel and booked them in at the reception desk. She picked up a key and handed it to Jean. 'You're sharing a bedroom on the first floor just up those stairs,' she stated, pointing to a flight of stairs to their left. 'I'll see you in the dining room, in a few minutes. It's down this corridor to the right,' she added, extending her arm towards it. You're okay with that, are you?' Jean nodded. She'd stayed with her parents in hotels and wasn't as nervous as Emma, with these strange surroundings.

'We'll be fine, thank you,' Jean replied. It was a short walk up the stairs to number twenty-five. Jean and Emma were obviously sharing a room on this first night with another young lady they had yet to meet, as there was already a suitcase by one of the beds. Emma was mesmerised by all that was happening.

After a quick wash and freshen up, the two girls made their way back downstairs to the dining room for the evening meal. On opening the door, a sea of faces met their gaze. Joan came forward to meet the girls and showed them to the remaining two empty chairs.

'There you are,' she said, pointing to the empty places. 'Bob, meet Emma and Jean from up North.' A tall, square-faced man with a stubbly, black beard flecked with grey, stood up and smiled.

'Welcome,' he said. The table was long and narrow with two adults towards one end and two nearer the other, with the youngsters, boys and girls of various ages, seated around. 'You've met Joan and Dot,' he continued, looking at Jean and Emma. 'They'll be going back to work tomorrow, but Tony,' he said, indicating a young, dark-haired male at the far end of the table, 'will be joining us for the whole trip. So, any questions, anytime and you can ask either Tony or myself.' Jean took the vacant chair next to Bob whilst Emma sat down near a young lad, about fourteen or fifteen, she guessed, who was on the other side of Jean and whose name, she learnt, was Martin.

As the food was being served by young waiters and waitresses, Bob tried to involve those around and opposite him, in conversation to counteract the silence and restraint. 'I know you'll all feel nervous and shy tonight,' he was saying, 'not knowing anyone. It's always like this at the first few meals but in a day or two you'll be laughing and joking like you've known each other for years.' He paused. 'Emma,' he said, turning towards her, 'tell us what it's like sheep rearing on your farm on the Yorkshire moors. What kind of sheep are they?' Emma hesitated for a moment whilst everyone around waited expectantly for her reply.
'Black-faced sheep, they're called. They're a hardy type, you know, because it's hilly with a lot of moorland and scrub, where I come from.' Emma wasn't sure if that was a correct answer, but she thought it sounded sensible enough and at least, she'd attempted some conversation which pleased her.

Throughout the course of the meal, everyone was asked something. Emma learnt that Martin came from Sheffield and she wondered how he'd become interested in farming. Opposite her was a freckled-faced boy called Kevin who appeared younger than her, she decided. He had a mop of ginger wavy hair and such a sweet, almost baby face with his snub nose. She studied Martin a little whilst he was listening to the girl opposite to him, who seemed loud-mouthed and noisy. The girl introduced herself as Gerry, short for Geraldine, she'd explained. Martin's hair was thick and wavy with a blond quiff at the front, stiff with brylcreem.

He caught Emma looking at him and winked. She blushed, feeling embarrassed and was glad when the meal finished.

They all trooped out and followed the staff to the common room where there was a television. Emma settled down in a very comfy chair to watch, as she'd never seen a television before although she knew one or two people in Windrush had them.
'First, we'll have to get electricity into Moorbeck,' she mused, 'and then money to buy one. I guess it'll be a while before that happens,' she concluded.
'Are you coming, Emma,' called Jean, a little later. 'I'm having an early night.' Emma, not wishing to stay around with people she didn't know, said a general good night as she left the common room and followed Jean upstairs. Later, when curled up in bed, resting her head on two very soft, luxurious pillows, she was thinking about the exciting day she'd had.
'I've loads to tell Martha when I get back home,' she thought, drifting off to sleep.

The next morning after breakfast, the party met in the lounge to have the day's agenda explained to them.
'The purpose of this Course,' stated Bob, 'whilst following the Severn river from its source to its mouth, is to contrast the farming and the farms and to meet the farmers to whom the Severn is their river. It won't all be hard work though. We want you to enjoy this experience. There will be lots of leisure time too. Today, we will be visiting a farm situated high up into the heart of Montgomeryshire and in sight of Plynlimon where the Severn has its source. It's in a very rural area. You will find the terrain rugged and hilly. We'll meet Mr Grayson at Staylittle who farms high up at one thousand, three hundred feet. Both the Hill Farming and Livestock Rearing Acts have enabled him with this government help, to rebuild his farmhouse and refurbish his farm buildings. Also, with draining, ploughing, pioneer cropping and reseeding, he has eventually trebled his Hereford herd as well as his hardy and picturesque flock of speckled-faced Kerries. Impressive. Kerries are a breed of sheep, by the way, in case some of you don't know. Kerry

Hill sheep originate from Kerry on the English/Welsh border. Hence the name.'

Bob checked his notes before continuing.
'On our second farm walk today, we'll descend to Llanidoes, rather lower by comparison at eight hundred and sixty feet but still hill farming. Here, at Cefn, we will meet Mr Wilson who has two hundred acres including forty acres of rough old bracken and woodland ready for improvement. The farm sustains over eighty head of cattle, Friesians and Welsh Black, but which are kept separately, you'll note, and a flock of sixty-six Kerry Hill ewes. Last spring, these sheep produced one hundred and seventeen lambs. I think you'll find it striking seeing lucerne flourishing at one thousand feet on boulder clay.
'What's lucerne?' a voice piped up. Emma looked around to see who was asking.
'It's Gerry, isn't it,' stated Bob, smiling at the girl who'd dared to ask. 'Well done for asking. It's always good to ask if you're unsure of something. Lucerne is a kind of grass used for grazing and for hay and silage. It's good stuff. I'm sure Mr Wilson will tell us more when you meet him today. So, plenty to take in. I hope you've all remembered your notebooks and pens or pencils as we will be meeting up tonight for a short period after dinner to discuss the farming methods we'll have seen today. Enjoy your trip. Your transport awaits,' he added, with a final flourish.

'Such a lot to take in,' thought Emma, who hadn't heard of some of the breeds of cattle and sheep. 'I must make lots of notes as I'll never remember all this stuff. I didn't know what lucerne was, either. I'm glad that girl asked.' The youngsters began chatting a little whilst jostling with each other as they scrambled for seats on the bus taking them on the long journey into Wales. Feeling relaxed and happy and enjoying the views that reminded her of the Yorkshire moors, Emma was enthusiastic and talkative on the bus, more so than some of her peers. Her laugh was infectious. It wasn't long before one or two of the others, becoming less nervous, were joining in with the banter. Emma took out her knitting from her bag. She'd asked Mary's advice about taking it and Mary pointed out that she might get quite a bit done whilst travelling on the buses. This was something of a surprise to the two members of staff, Bob and Tony, but they decided that if it was put away before dismounting the bus, they couldn't see any objections. Most of the youngsters found it strange too.

The day passed quickly and included some quite strenuous walking but without any hiccups. Everyone seemed to be writing copious notes along the way. After the exhausting walk around the second farm, there was an unexpected delight for the party when invited into the farmhouse kitchen to a spread of cakes and scones, prepared for them by Mrs Wilson, plus as much tea as they could drink. Later in the evening, after returning to the hotel and following supper, there was a rendezvous in the Assembly Rooms where Tony and Bob instigated a good natter over the events of the day, although at this stage, Emma noticed that the young people were mostly too shy to ask questions.
'Maybe I'll ask one tomorrow night,' she thought, before dropping off to sleep.

The next day was equally packed with activity. The first farm the party visited belonged to Major Hall who explained that although his farm, situated on the Severn shore beside Newtown, was under forty acres, its excellent grass feed meant that five hundred gallons of milk were produced per acre. The Grassland Officer for Wales made an appearance. Everyone was invited to go on all fours to explore and name, if possible, the many varieties of grass.

Lunch consisted of sandwiches and a local brew of pop, partaken whilst the bus continued to a Severn farm, lower Mr Griffin, a celebrated farmer, was keen to show everyone his Kerry sheep and Shorthorn cattle, before taking the group inside to another wonderful spread of eats and to show the silver cup that he'd won outright for three consecutive years. He also explained that the name of his farm, Gaer, meant camp, as it was situated on the site of an old Roman fortress.
'We will be stopping on the way back,' Bob interjected, 'near Offa's dyke, the rampart thrown up in the ninth century to mark the division between Wales and the kingdom of

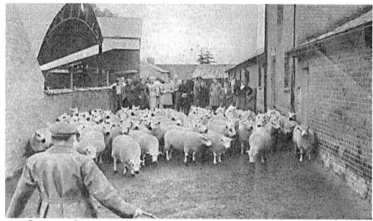

Severn Course – Admiring prize-winning Kerry sheep

Mercia.' He paused and glanced around to see if the young people were following, before adding, 'and after that, the Severn we follow will be babbling in English.' This comment produced a few grins and he knew he was being listened to. 'It's all such great fun,' thought Emma, 'and with meals prepared and no washing up.' The two years at boarding school, although it was an all-girls school, gave her an edge over some of the other girls on this trip who were having to adjust to mixing with other youngsters, both throughout the day and in the evenings. Also, having an older brother added to her experience, as she was used to being teased by Tim. All this enabled her to have more confidence in mixing than some of the party, who were still a little subdued and less at ease. She didn't even mind the teasing by one or two of them.

There were some sleepy heads next morning at breakfast and not much conversation. A rather long and sometimes hilarious discussion the previous evening, the group becoming more at ease with one another, added to the tiredness of the hectic day. This meant a late night and a reluctance to rise early.
'Good morning, everyone,' announced Tony, looking at the serious faces, whilst brushing his rather unkempt, long hair from his face. 'A great session last night. Thank you for participating so well. Another full day today, though. This

morning we meet a young farmer, Mr Mosey, at Lea Hill farm and he shares his dad's belief in organics. It will be a fascinating learning curve for most of us, including me I'm sure, as I know little about organic farming, but I'm looking forward to it. Then after lunch we're visiting Longford Grange and, as you'll find out, it is a very mechanised farm. Here, there will be two specialists, as well as our host, Mr Bowman, to answer all the questions you can drum up, about the various machinery we will be shown. You will be pleased to know that transport is being arranged to take us around his farm. Not the usual kind, of course, but I'm sure you will enjoy it. Don't forget we move to another hotel this evening. Make sure you bring your bags to the bus after breakfast. Enjoy your day.'

'It sounds great,' Emma said to Jean, sitting next to her. 'It's all so different to our farm. Ours is so basic I suppose.'
'It's not what I'm used to either. I know plenty about turkey rearing but not much else.'
'Tony was right,' Emma decided later, that learning about organic farming was fascinating, but the ride around the second farm on a trailer was the highlight for her. There was plenty to interest everyone as the tractor chugged its way across the rough tracks. 'I never knew such farming machinery existed,' she thought, on watching the grass drying machine gorging on lucerne. This piece of machinery went from farm to farm, they were told, 'a bit like the threshing machine does at home,' thought Emma, 'but here they have combine harvesters as well. Maybe one day,' she mused, 'and it must save a lot of hard graft, as her dad would say.'

Early in the evening, the bus pulled up outside what Emma thought looked like a rather grand hotel. They'd arrived at Dodington on the southern outskirts of Whitchurch. Climbing down from the bus after Jean, Emma followed her through the revolving doors of the hotel and into the reception area. 'Gosh,' thought Emma, gazing around at the large, comfortable chairs with their burgundy, plush upholstery and noticing the gleaming, wooden furniture. 'Very posh,' she thought, enjoying the lush sensation of her shoes sinking into the dark grey carpet. Bob was already at reception signing in the party and handing out keys. A young man, very smartly dressed in his pin-striped grey suit, crisp white shirt and burgundy-coloured tie, came over to speak with them.

'I'll show you to your room,' the young man explained to Jean and Emma as they were at the front of the queue, whilst taking their luggage from them. 'Just follow me, please.'

'He's a porter,' explained Jean to Emma, noticing Emma's anxious face when he took her case. 'It's their job to carry our luggage.'

'Fancy his tie matching the colour of the chairs,' Emma thought, walking behind him and wondering if it was deliberate. They went with him into a lift with others of their party crowding in, after them.

The lift stopped at the second floor, the doors slid open and they all stepped outside onto thick-piled speckled maroon and grey carpet. The porter led Jean and Emma to a bedroom halfway down the long corridor, opened the door for them and placed their luggage on the carpet inside.

'Thank you,' the two girls chorused, as he left.

'Wonder who is joining us?' said Jean, looking at the four beds. Then the door opened and Gerry walked in.

'Hi, I'm with you three now. I'll have this bed,' Gerry said to them, jumping onto the one nearest the window. Emma smiled politely, in acknowledgement, although she wasn't very keen on Gerry. She started to unpack.

'Did you know,' stated Gerry, 'that in this hotel, if you put your shoes outside the door at night, the next morning, they will have been cleaned for you?'

'Really?' said Emma, in amazement, trying to be a little friendly. 'I might try that tonight,' she stated, not thinking it would happen. They settled in and wandered down to the dining room for the evening meal, after which, the photographer who accompanied the trips to take photos for The Farmers Weekly, put on a film show, a welcome change from farming discussions.

Awakening early next morning, Emma crawled out of bed and went to check on her shoes.

'It's true,' she thought, quite amazed on examining her

beautifully polished shoes. 'Fancy that,' she exclaimed, on re-entering the bedroom and seeing the other three girls awake. 'Just look at my shoes.'
'See, I told you,' Gerry bragged. On arriving in the dining room for breakfast, Emma had barely sat down when Martin sidled up to the empty chair on Emma's left. He'd taken quite an interest in Emma and she'd reciprocated, enjoying his company. He was following close behind when she was stepping onto the bus and Emma knew he'd try to sit with her.

'More knitting, Emma?' asked Bob, with a twinkle in his eye, as she climbed on. Emma grinned and nodded. She looked around before taking the empty seat next to Kevin and smiling at him, she sat down, leaving Martin to go elsewhere. It was a long uphill ride on single track roads, over brooklets and cattle grids, until at one thousand and one hundred feet, the party arrived at the farm of Mr Cousin. From there, they could see mile upon mile of valley and beyond that, the ridge of Longmynd. Mr Cousin worked two hundred and seventy acres of marshy hill land in conjunction with a lowland farm of four hundred and sixty acres, some twenty miles away. It was quite isolated up on the hill farm

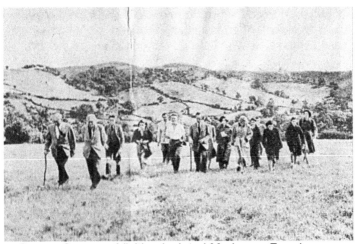

Severn Course – Visiting isolated Marhayes Farmhouse

and intrepid for the tractor drivers on the steep slopes. The rain came down as they journeyed back to the hotel, but Emma was happily knitting whilst thinking of those cattle grids. She thought they would be a great idea for her dad. 'Save opening and shutting all the gates in and out of Moorbeck,' she surmised.

As breakfast was finishing the following morning, Bob rose from his chair, wiping his mouth on his serviette before placing it at the side of his plate. He gazed around at the youngsters, waiting for a lull in the chattering, before making his announcement.

'Today, we do something different.' The noise around the table subsided as everyone waited to hear what was next. 'We're going to visit Wroxeter where Watling Street crosses the Severn. You will get a lot of history from our guide today as we will hear how the Romans took five years to reach the Severn from their landing in Kent with their Emperor Claudius in August AD 43. They built a camp and settled down for twenty-five years before moving up country to Chester. Anyway, I'll leave it there as you'll learn more during our tour although there's not much left to see in the way of ruins. Then, this afternoon, we're going to the pictures. That, you will enjoy,' he added, with a grin. 'If any of you want to go to church tomorrow, have a word with Tony or myself. Apart from that, it's a free day. Maybe catch up on some sleep,' he finished, smiling at the youngsters.

Over the last day or two, as well as enjoying Martin's attention, Emma had found herself becoming quite friendly with Kevin. She learnt that he was the youngest competitor on this trip and a year younger than herself. She found him to be a gentle and kind lad, quiet and shy. Maybe it was his baby face that reminded her of her younger brother, Mark, she thought. She made a point of chatting to him, enjoying his company whilst feeling a little motherly towards him.

Whatever activity was happening, either in the hotels or out on their excursions, Emma observed that some of the older ones were eyeing each other up, one fancying another, as adolescents do. It was obvious that Gerry was wanting to be noticed by the tall, good-looking Martin and whenever possible, edged her way into his company. It was also plain to see that Martin was showing an interest in Emma. Her awareness of boys was growing. She knew he was trying to get her attention. Emma, flattered by this, teased and plagued him just as she would her older brother Tim. They sparred a little when meeting up. She enjoyed the banter. The adults, supervising this mixed bunch of youngsters, were highly amused at times, but other times had to quietly speak with them if they were too boisterous in the hotels. By Sunday evening, everyone was relaxed and friendly with earlier reservations blown away.

'It's great to see how much you're enjoying yourselves,' said Bob, on Sunday at the end of the evening meal, 'but please can you keep your noise level down a little. Other people are staying here too.'

It was a weekend of fun for Emma and she caught up on her note writing too. Not everyone, however, enjoyed her mischievous ways as she found out when she was preparing for bed on Sunday evening. Jean was already in bed, quietly reading. Gerry, the loudly spoken girl was talking to Melanie, who was seventeen and the oldest of all the winners and sharing the bedroom with them. Emma was the youngest of the four. Melanie, tall, blond and seemingly to Emma, a little snooty, found Emma's lively spirit difficult to cope with, having already shared a bedroom with her at the previous hotel.

'Have you really put a worm into my bed?' she demanded to know, sitting on a chair in her thin cotton, floral pyjamas.

'Of course I haven't,' said Emma, grinning from ear to ear. 'I wouldn't do a thing like that.'

Earlier, Martin had been chasing her around the garden of the hotel threatening to put a worm down the back of her tee-shirt. She'd bumped into Melanie and jokingly said that if he did, she was going to put it in Melanie's bed. She'd remembered Martha once playing this trick on her, pretending she would do such a thing and how annoying it was, not being sure whether she would do it. Emma didn't intend to, but Melanie felt irritated and uncertain about Emma telling the truth. Consequently, Melanie refused to sleep in her own bed.

'Honestly, Emma. You are a pest. You can sleep in my bed tonight.' Emma grinned.

'Okay. Fine,' she said. 'There is nothing in yours. I was only joking.'

'Nevertheless, I'm not risking it,' stated Melanie, walking over to Emma's bed. Emma didn't mind. She thought they were all too serious.

'It is a holiday,' she thought. 'Holidays are for fun.'

The familiarity of the youngsters was evident on the bus journey on Monday morning, a total contrast from the first Monday. Some broke into song, whilst on the long back seat, others played an ambiguous game of forfeits. One or two entertained with stories. Emma was a little embarrassed when Martin sat down beside her and took her knitting pattern and began reading out loud the instructions, much to the amusement of the leaders and some of the girls and boys. Emma took this in good spirit but was secretly planning to play a joke on Martin after the incident with the worm at the weekend.

'Did you know about getting your shoes cleaned at night?' she questioned him. 'You just try it. Leave them outside your door. It worked for me.' She was devising a plan in her head, but she wasn't telling anyone. 'I'll wait a day or so before I carry it out,' she decided, thinking of the mischief she intended. The following morning after breakfast, Emma caught up with Martin. 'Did you ever leave your shoes out to be cleaned,' she asked him, as they were stepping onto the bus.

'I did, and it worked,' he answered. Emma smiled, knowingly.

'Maybe tonight,' she thought.

Meanwhile, it was another long journey moving southwards and never far from the Severn's influence, but eventually, the party arrived at Leominster in Herefordshire. Mr Coats was very informative about his occupation of breeding, exhibiting and judging Shorthorn cattle. After he explained the good points of a Shorthorn when judging, there was plenty of fun for the youngsters in giving points on a group of heifers, at his invitation. An interesting sight was a flock of Muscovy ducks that roosted on the roof-tops and being

warned by Mr Coats of their terrifying habits of low-flying.
'A long but enjoyable day,' thought Emma, as the bus pulled
into the hotel's car park.

It was very early the following morning, on the pretext of
going to the toilet, that Emma crept quietly down the
corridor. Most of The Farmers Weekly party were on this
floor and the youngsters visited each other in the bedrooms
sometimes whilst waiting to go downstairs for the evening
meal and feedback from the day. She spied Martin's black
shoes, polished and shiny, outside his bedroom door. She
took from her dressing gown pocket, a tube of toothpaste
and reaching into the toe of each shoe, she squeezed some
out. She very quickly scurried back along to her bedroom,
smiling to herself.
'That'll pay him back for teasing and chasing me with the
worm,' she thought, happily.

Later, at breakfast, Emma refused to meet Martin's gaze. He
was a little late for breakfast and was seated at the next
table, but she heard him raise his voice as he stated that if
anyone was running out of toothpaste, they were welcome to
borrow his. Emma concentrated on eating, not daring to look
over at him, wondering that maybe, she'd gone too far with
her little trick. Later, when they were all walking to the bus
parked at the end of the car park, Martin brushed passed
her.
'Just you wait and see what'll happen,' he whispered. He
caught up with Gerry and began chatting to her, much to
Gerry's delight.
'She's only a kid,' she heard Gerry say to Martin, well within
earshot of Emma who was climbing onto the bus, after them.
'That's what she thinks, is it?' questioned Emma, to herself.
'I think she's just putting me down because she is jealous.'

It turned out to be another day of great interest to Emma
after a delightful drive over the Malvern Hills down across
the widening Severn and up to a Cotswold farm beyond
Cheltenham where Mr Rowan was waiting to greet the party.
He owned a total of one hundred and sixty Friesian cattle
which produced over one thousand gallons of milk on
average. The milking parlour was unlike anything Emma

could even imagine. Mr Rowan demonstrated the workings of the gates, portcullises and traps whereby each cow is guided to the teat-cups. As it was between milking times, he made do with half a dozen heifers, shuffling them around as in a maze, while he controlled the works which finally imprisoned them in tandem. The youngsters were fascinated, not having seen anything as modern as this before.

'It must cost a fortune,' thought Emma.

Mr Rowan continued the tour explaining about his three to four thousand head of poultry which the party observed, from seeing new-laid eggs to the unusual sight of some hens walking around wearing plastic spectacles. Mr Rowan was keen to explain that they clap the glasses onto the feathers of certain egg-pecking hens to prevent them from damaging the eggs. Although production was intense right through from incubation, he was reassuring in that the hens happily enjoyed outdoor summer pasture.

It was a long day for the youngsters and staff, but a very educational one studying the modern farming methods. After evening meal, there was a question and answer session to see just how much the young people had learnt, following which, Emma went to her bedroom. She was very tired and next morning, was late getting out of bed as she was still sleepy. She dressed quickly and went to retrieve her shoes from outside the bedroom door. Some of the boys and girls were already making their way along the corridor to go down to breakfast.

'Oh, no!' exclaimed Emma as she placed her foot inside the shoe. Something was very wrong. She brought her foot out. The toe end of her sock was covered in a mess. It was brylcreem. 'It's what Tim uses for his hair, sometimes,' she thought. 'Well, I guess I asked for it,' she mused, realising that Martin was getting his revenge. She removed her sock and found a clean pair but spent time cleaning the inside of her shoes. Consequently, she was late for breakfast.

'Not like you to be late,' commented Tony. 'Still tired after the long day, yesterday, are you?' Emma nodded sheepishly and took the only remaining empty seat which happened to be directly opposite Martin. He smiled at her and then, turning to his nearest neighbour, asked loudly, 'You don't happen to have any brylcreem to spare, do you, as I seem to have run short.' He glanced back at Emma, winking at her, but she ignored him and concentrated on her breakfast.

Emma made a point of avoiding Martin and staying around Kevin during their day on another farm on the farther side of Gloucester on the outskirts of Dursley. This time, although it was more Cotswold farming, it was totally different from yesterday's farm. This one was situated between industry and woodland and Mr Prudom explained the damage done to his crops by both trespassers and by badgers. As well as working his farmland, he ran a retail milk round with the milk from his farm mainly from Friesians but as he explained, with a lacing of Guernseys to give the milk that touch of colour which the customers believed was good for them. His little dairy was extremely well scrubbed, very competent and mechanised as to the sterilising, bottling and capping. 'It's amazing,' thought Emma, 'and fascinating to see at first hand, how the milk ends up bottled ready for sale.' She added Guernsey to her list of cattle breeds learnt on these trips.

The party walked the length of the farm before returning to their bus. It had been another well planned and busy day, which Emma enjoyed. Kevin, being painfully shy, was undemanding and Emma enjoyed the peaceful atmosphere and calmness. She was more subdued than usual, but Kevin was happy to be in her company. They'd quietly talked or made notes and he even chatted a little about his home life.

'Can we have a bit of quiet, please,' requested Tony, above the rattle of pots and cutlery. It was breakfast, the following morning and the youngsters paused in their chatter, waiting with expectation for the announcement. Tony, standing at one end of their long table, was looking at his notes. 'Just to warn you that a television cameraman is joining us today. Yes, that's right,' he added, looking at their surprised expressions. The Farmers Weekly want a short piece recorded that will eventually go out nationally on television on the Children's Newsreel programme. The cameraman will be covering you watching the cheese-making process, Cheddar cheese, that is. I'm sure you've all heard of it. This area is well known for its Cheddar cheese. Just carry on as normal, though and enjoy the day.' There was a buzz of excitement among the youngsters when this was announced, with the expectation of being on camera. The noise continued as they wandered out of the dining room in twos and threes.

Later in the morning, the party arrived at Mr Ainthorp's farm at Langford in Somerset, to be met not only by him but by a cameraman, pointing his lens at the file of youngsters and adults stepping from the bus and continuing with his shoot as they walked down the lane. Arriving at the farm buildings,

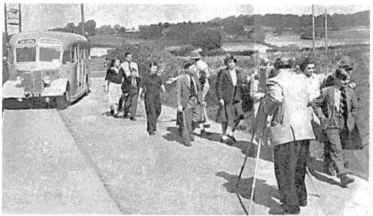

Severn Course – Arriving at the cheese-making farm

they gathered around Mr Ainthorp who enthused over his farm, explaining that cheese and bacon were its mainstays with all the milk being made into cheese and the whey pumped into the piggeries. They followed him into a building where the process of cheese-making was underway, crowding around to watch for themselves. Emma was fascinated, looking at the whey running off and then the cutting into blocks of the white spongy solids. She continued watching as the workers lifted the blocks of curds from the trough.

'Now, a closeup of three of you,' announced the cameraman, who'd been occupied filming the process and the onlookers. The girls and boys looked at each other, not knowing who he meant. 'We'll have you,' he continued, pointing to Jean. 'You with the curly black hair,' he added, looking at Emma. 'Then we'll have the ginger-haired lad. Right, all three of you stand closer to this empty cheese trough. Don't look at the camera or lights. What's your name, laddie?' he asked.

'Kevin.'

'I want you, Kevin, to stand between the girls and point your finger as if you're describing something in the trough and you girls look to where he's pointing. Don't look at me. Okay?' They nodded.

The camera rolled and Emma, with a serious expression on her face, followed intently the direction of Kevin's finger, as if she was totally engrossed, even though there was nothing to see. It was all over in seconds but as they were being filmed, Emma heard Martin behind her, commenting in a slightly raised voice and with a touch of sarcasm, intending for her to hear.

'Look well together, don't they?' As she turned around, she noticed that he was speaking to Gerry.

'He's missing my jokes and fun,' she thought. 'He's just trying to make me feel uncomfortable. Maybe I shouldn't have done that with his shoes. He's quite nice really.'

The afternoon was spent at Mr Martin's farm at Tetbury after they'd journeyed back to the Cotswolds through Bristol. This was a traditional farm where not only were sheep reared and fattened on a large scale but also the farmer ran a herd of beef cattle comprising a mix of Hereford pure, Hereford-Shorthorn and Hereford-Friesian. Mr Martin led the party on foot to a stretch of stone wall where he explained a little about the art that goes into stonewalling. As they all clambered onto the bus at the end of the day, Martin made sure he was sitting next to Emma and with gentle teasing, managed to persuade her to talk with him. There followed the evening meal with another film show, a most instructive supplement to the outdoor observations, although Tony and Bob were a little bemused at the motor-racing one that casually was slipped in between Grass-Drying and Care of Livestock.

The holiday, as Emma thought of it, even though very instructive, was coming to an end.
'Only one more full day,' she mused, ticking off another date on her small calendar. This last day was spent at Somerset Farm Institute at Cannington on the far side of Bridgewater and with a seaside lunch at Weston-Super-Mare. Again, Martin spent most of the time, when possible, in Emma's company and she enjoyed the attention. The Principal of the Institute, whilst unable to be with them, had arranged a varied programme that amounted to an agricultural education in miniature, by the heads of the horticulture, dairying and crop husbandry departments. The youngsters also inspected the poultry, the market garden crops and blue pigs. They even compared the cheese-making with that of Mr Ainthorp's, the day before.

As Bob and Tony mingled with their party and after listening to the many intelligent questions put by the youngsters, they realised just how much they'd learnt.
'You know, Bob,' commented Tony, as they straggled behind the young adults walking towards the bus for the final time, 'it's been well worth it, hasn't it, when you hear how they responded with their questions today. They've learnt a lot and so have I. We've seen so much with great input from farmers and others and travelled over a thousand miles. Not often, if ever, one gets an opportunity to see such a variety of farming and the different terrains in less than two weeks.'
Bob nodded. He was tired and ready for home.

On this last night, Emma and a group of boys and girls were chatting pleasantly in the bedroom that she shared with Jean, Melanie and Gerry. One by one, they drifted out to go downstairs for the evening meal until only Jean, Martin and Emma remained. Emma was full of excitement at going home and in high spirits. She'd been teasing Martin yet again, not realising that a fifteen-year old boy can be quite fascinated but also frustrated by such attention. Emma was sitting on the edge of her bed, swinging her legs backwards and forwards, when, suddenly, Martin moved across to her,

140

pushing her onto her back on the bed and whilst pinning her arms down, kissed her a couple of times on her cheek. Emma was surprised and shocked as she's never been kissed by a young man before. Adding to this, she was embarrassed as Jean was watching with a bemused look on her face. Emma struggled to get up. Martin immediately released her and ran out of the room. It was all over in seconds, but Emma was a mixture of emotions and felt a little angry and upset.

'Come on,' said Jean, watching Emma. 'He's harmless. He just likes you, that's all. Let's go down to eat.'

Arriving in the dining room, Emma deliberately avoided Martin, making sure that she was seated away from his table. After dinner, the party convened as usual but confined this, their last get-together, to a round-up of the last two weeks and agreeing what fun it had been. Melanie, being the eldest, expressed the thanks of them all to The Farmers Weekly staff for arranging the course, to which Bob responded and asked them what they'd liked best as a help in planning future courses. The youngsters were eager in giving their opinions and reminiscences on such an interesting and educational few days they'd experienced and enjoyed so much. When the conversation was beginning to verge on sentimentality, Bob brought the gathering to a close. He whispered to Tony.

'Fancy a pint at the bar?' Tony grinned and nodded.

At breakfast, next morning, the atmosphere was rather subdued.

'It's been such an amazing time,' said Emma to Kevin, sitting beside her. He smiled and nodded. 'Such a sweet boy,' she thought. She was still feeling a little nervous of meeting with Martin and was deliberately keeping her distance. Then Joan, who'd arrived late the previous evening and joined Tony and Bob at the bar for a long chat about the two weeks, got up from her chair, tapping her spoon on the table to gain attention whilst waiting for the chattering to cease.

'Hello again, everyone. I hear you've had a great time. Bob and Tony filled me in last night. I have travel arrangements for you.' She went through each name, checking and making sure that every competitor was happy about their journey. 'Emma, you will travel with Martin as far as Sheffield, but you remain on the train to York from where you can catch a bus to Whitby. I have spoken with your dad who telephoned me. He reassured me that you are familiar with the remainder of your journey home from Whitby. One of our representative's will meet you off the train at York and see you safely on the bus. Just hold up your Farmers Weekly. Okay?' Emma nodded, her heart sinking a little. She felt unsure of Martin now. She glanced up at him only to find him looking at her. He gave her a gentle smile and put his thumb up.

'Maybe it'll be okay,' she thought. 'He can't do much on a train full of people.'

'Finally,' continued Joan, 'there are packed lunches on the side table for those on long journeys. You can pick one up on your way out. Likewise, for those travelling by train, the tickets are there too. I hope you all have a safe journey. Don't forget to watch Children's Newsreel. I will let you know which week is scheduled to broadcast our trip, as soon as I find out.'

There were many farewells and even a few hugs, as the young people, in ones and twos, made their get-a-ways. Jean was going a different route to visit an aunt whilst this far down the country and her mother was joining her. Martin and Emma shared a taxi to the station with others going their way. Then Emma followed Martin to the platform. He was quieter than usual, but they made small talk until the train pulled into the platform.

'I'll take that,' he said, picking up her case. They sat side by side on the crowded train and eventually, after some hesitation from both, they began talking with ease, each enjoying these last few hours together after very many eventful days.

'Sorry about the toothpaste,' Emma finally admitted. 'I got a bit carried away.'

'Me too, with the brylcreem. Let's forget it. I'm glad I've met you, Emma. You're such fun. Maybe you'll write to me,' he replied, hesitantly, his blond hair falling loosely over his brow. 'This is my address if you want to tell me how you're doing. Boarding school sounds fascinating.' Emma smiled. 'Thanks,' she said, taking the slip of paper and putting it in

her purse. 'I might do that.'
'Sheffield next stop,' Martin said. 'It has been great these few days, Emma and maybe we'll meet again. You're sweet, you know,' he added, shyly, not knowing quite how to leave. Then he stood up as the train pulled into the station, and taking his case from the rack, walked down the gangway and off the train. Seeing him standing looking at the train as she gazed through the window, Emma smiled and waved, watching Martin waving back until he was no longer visible. 'Well,' she sighed, feeling a little emotional and mixed-up and wondering what she'd tell Martha. 'Maybe I won't tell all of it and certainly not to mam and dad.'

On her arrival home, the family plagued Emma for details of her adventure and she explained many of the excursions but little about her encounters with Martin. She showed no-one his address but copied it into her diary and burnt the piece of paper. She was feeling flat after such an exhilarating experience with so many memories and thoughts of the days spent with the prize winners. A week later, a letter arrived from The Farmers Weekly giving details of the forthcoming broadcast of the filming of cheese-making. It was to be shown on the five o'clock Children's Newsreel programme on Friday, the eleventh of September. Mary wasn't over-enthusiastic when hearing about this, as they didn't have a television but knew that Emma might like to see it.
'You could walk down to Mrs Hartness in the village, as she has recently bought a television. She was telling us, after Mass, all about the programmes she can see on the little box, as she calls it. I'll ask her on Sunday if you like. I'm sure she won't mind. You could take Martha with you. It's good that you don't go back to school till the sixteenth, otherwise you would have missed it.'
'That would be great. I'd love that,' replied Emma. 'You'll come with me, won't you, Martha?' Martha nodded.

On Monday afternoon, the two girls set off with plenty of time and tramped the mile over the moor and another on the road to the village. It was a hot summer's day. They arrived at the village green which was surrounded by a semi-circle of houses. Walking across to the far corner and undoing the latch on a wooden gate, they went down the pebble-covered path to a blue door.

'Come in, lasses,' invited Mrs Hartness, when she opened the door to them. 'I've been expecting you. You'll be wanting a drink after your long walk in this heat.' She was a little stout lady, quite elderly and a motherly type of person whom Emma often saw at church. She had curly grey hair and wore thick-framed glasses. She showed the girls into her front room and went to the kitchen, returning with glasses of orange squash. 'There you are. Take a seat. I'll just turn the television on,' she said, moving to the small box that was placed on a stand in the corner of the room. Emma noticed how neat and tidy the room was, with plumped up cushions on comfortable chairs and polished surfaces covered with plants, ornaments and photographs.

Then her attention turned to the television.

'Fascinating,' she thought, watching the pictures flit across the screen and listening to the speakers. 'Amazing,' she kept thinking. Although she'd watched television at the hotel when on her trip, she was still almost spellbound at viewing one here in their own village. Her ears pricked up at the introduction to the news item that they'd come to see. 'Look,' she said. 'That's us.' The prize winners were chattering and smiling as they walked down the lane. 'Oh, my,' she exclaimed, as the short news piece continued. 'There will be a close-up of just three of us, any minute now.' Then the shot of the faces of Jean, Kevin and Emma, concentrating on looking at a trough supposedly full of cheese, filled the screen.

'Emma, you do suit that hair style. Very grown-up, you know,' said Mrs Hartness, smiling at Emma, before turning her gaze back to the screen. It was all over in seconds, it seemed, but not before Emma spotted Martin in a group shot.

'He is good looking,' she thought. 'I think I might write to him when I get back to school.'

The girls said thanks to Mrs Hartness and set off up the village back home.

'Fancy being on television,' commented Martha. 'You didn't look up, though, at the camera, I mean.'

'We were told not to, by the cameraman man.'

'But it was quite easy to see who you were,' Martha added, reassuringly. 'I wonder if anyone else recognised you.'
Emma was wondering, too, especially thinking about her peers at school.
'What will they make of it,' she mused, 'and the nuns too, if they saw it. Me on television.' Emma could hardly believe it.

Autumn to Summer 1954

'Look at your hair. You've had it permed,' said Maria, thinking of her own mouse-coloured hair, straight and short with a fringe at the front. Emma was on the bus, walking up to the back row, joining the girls returning to boarding school. 'It looks good, Emma. Makes you look older too. I bet you're taller than me now.' It was a similar response from Faith, later in the evening.

'I think you really suit your hair, Emma. It makes you look more grown-up. Did your mam do it for you? Someone on our table at supper mentioned that they'd seen you on television. Is that true? Was it to do with your prize when you went away? I'm dying to hear about it. Were there any interesting boys on it?' she questioned, as she, too, was beginning to take an interest in lads. Emma nodded and grinned, feeling her face redden.

'Yes, my mam gave me and Martha home perms. The television people came one day and took shots of us when we were on the trip,' Emma continued. She was still relating the highlights of her thirteen days away when the noise of the bell interrupted their conversation. 'More later,' she whispered to Faith as the girls lined up in silence to go to the dormitories.

There was a similar reaction about her hair when a much more confident Emma, than in her first two years, walked into the form room the next morning. She'd held her high position, never coming below fifth. This gave Emma immense satisfaction and helped to counteract her concerns over her lack of general knowledge and different background.

'We've been talking about you,' Peg stated. 'Some of us saw you on television. You kept that quiet. When did all that happen and why?' The other pupils stopped talking, listening to this conversation.

'Well, I didn't know until the summer holidays, that I'd won,' explained Emma.

'You've had your hair done as well,' Peg continued. 'It suits you.'

'Thank you. My mam gave me a home perm and my sister too.' She continued with her story until the door opened and a teacher walked in. She'd accompanied them from the assembly hall to the form room, but then left after formally introducing herself. Miss Watson was one of the newly appointed teachers from university. As well as being their form teacher, she would be taking them for Geography and occasionally for some PE lessons. Not having known Emma, Miss Watson made no comment on her television appearance.

It was later in the morning, when it was referred to again by the nun in charge at recreation after dinner. Outside in the convent grounds, some pupils were practising tennis whilst others were standing in groups catching up on holidays. Emma was sitting on one of the benches with her nose in a book when she was aware that someone was speaking to her.
'I hear we have a star in our presence,' the nun said, on approaching Emma. Some of the girls within earshot, stopped to listen. Emma reddened. She felt embarrassed.
'It was a competition run by The Farmers Weekly that I won along with a number of others,' Emma explained. She continued talking, choosing her words carefully and trying to play down her appearance on television.
'And those eyebrows, do you put something on them?' the questioning continued with the nun looking at Emma's thick, black, curved eyebrows. Emma shook her head, very surprised at this personal question.
'I've always had these eyebrows,' she stated, not knowing what else to say. 'I don't do anything to them.' The nun tutted and wandered off. Emma returned to her book, not enjoying the attention nor the giggles from the onlookers.

Speaking about the trip reminded Emma of Martin and she decided that she would write to him. She wondered about how to get a letter posted and decided that she'd ask Laura if she could do that, as Emma wasn't sure about handing it in at Saturday letter writing time. Mother Colette might spot it, she thought. It was a surprise at the beginning of this term when, instead of Mother Monica, Mother Colette was greeting the boarders outside the dormitory when they'd first arrived, with a smile on her face and her blue eyes twinkling. She was not as tall as her predecessor but almost as slim under her long, black clothes.

'She must be a teacher,' thought Emma, noticing the blue cloth hanging down the front.

'She seems very pleasant, doesn't she,' stated Faith, later in the evening, when catching up with Emma at recreation.

'She does. Less stern-looking and formidable but maybe that's me feeling less in awe of them.' However, Emma wasn't sure how Mother Colette would react if she left the letter to Martin to be posted with the others. She was confident that Laura wouldn't tell on her as she kept to herself a lot. After joining Emma in the very small parts in the play the previous school year, she always seemed happy speaking with her when needing advice about homework.

Later that evening, snuggled up in bed with her cubicle curtain drawn, Emma took out her cheap note pad and began writing a letter to Martin. She'd been delighted when returning to school for the autumn term, to find that she'd been allocated a cubicle on the street side of the dormitory. It was noisy, with the occupants of the junior dormitory walking up and down the corridor as well as from the traffic below on the street, but a great improvement from being in the junior dormitory and much more private. It was dark before she'd written much, having restarted the letter numerous times. The letter remained unfinished for many weeks until Emma finally drafted one that she was happy with and asked Laura to post it, whilst wondering if Martin would write back. She'd put her home address on as she wasn't sure how Mother Colette would react, when handing out the post, seeing a different writing style on the envelope, if Martin ever wrote back.

'Don't tell anyone, will you?' she asked. Laura smiled.

'Of course I won't. I've met a lad I'm seeing occasionally but I don't talk about it here. Your secret's safe with me.'

There were other advantages to being in a cubicle, Emma realised, one of which was to do with laundry. Emma's white ankle socks became scruffy very quickly and slack around the tops where she turned them over. She usually made them last days in the junior dormitory as she didn't have many pairs. Now she hand-washed them with her soap in the basin in her cubicle and hung them on the metal bar

underneath where they eventually dried.
'They're not exactly crisp and white,' she mused, 'but they are cleaner and fold over more neatly. I can change them more often too.'

Emma didn't hear from Martin until the Christmas holidays, when he sent her a Christmas card and wrote a short note inside saying how much he'd enjoyed receiving her letter. Emma was quite thrilled and shared her thoughts with Martha, finally telling her about the goings-on, on the trip. When the card arrived, Mary didn't ask questions about it, which Emma thought unusual. Emma didn't tell her mam that she'd written first, not that her mam would have been bothered, she thought, as Mary seemed pre-occupied over Christmas and a little edgy and tired. She didn't want to go to the dance at Windrush, either, much to the girls' surprise. Emma asked if Faith might come for a stay, but Mary said that Christmas was a bit busy and that Faith might want to be with her sister and uncles at such a time.
'Another time,' she said to Emma.

There was some good news though. After milking, when Tom was settled in for the evening and they were playing a game of whist with him and Tim, he asked them a question.
'Do you lasses want to go dancing tomorrow night? Jack Netherfield says he'll pick us up. Tim isn't bothered, are you Tim?' Tim shook his head. Emma's eyes lit up.
'I'd love to.'
'That'll be great,' Martha stated. 'I'll help you, Emma, to find something to wear. You're almost as tall as me now.' She looked at her dad and grinned.
'Aye, I know; he might be there,' he laughed, guessing his daughter's thoughts. He'd seen Martha's reaction to the lad at their neighbour's farm, High Acres, when they'd visited recently. Martha blushed. His reply was exactly what she was hoping for.

Before Jack Netherfield arrived the following evening, Tom called to his two older daughters who were in their downstairs bedroom. He stood in the passageway and closed the kitchen door so that no-one else could hear him.
'You lasses need to know this,' he said. 'You've probably

been wondering about Jack Netherfield. You may hear rumours from the village folk when you're at the dance. So, I'm telling you first. I'm not going into details as there's no need, but I want you know that he's my brother and your uncle. Strictly speaking, he's my half-brother, a month or so older than me. My dad is his dad. So, if anyone one says anything tonight, just tell them you know and change the subject. Tim knows, but don't mention it to the little ones as they don't know yet.'

The girls looked at each other, meaningfully and at their dad. They were both gobsmacked. They'd thought there was a resemblance. They'd talked about it, with Mr Netherfield being so friendly to the family and guessed right about maybe him being a relative of their dad's, but a brother! Their real uncle! 'You needn't mention it to Jack unless you want to as I'll tell him I've told you. He's been wanting you to know, for some time. Here he is now,' he concluded, hearing the coals door open. The girls said hello to Jack and went out to climb into the back of the van without mentioning this latest news. The two brothers talked farming in the front, whilst the girls chatted quietly, sitting on the van floor that was covered with empty sacks.

The dance lived up to Emma's expectation. There were teenagers and adults including some mams and dads. The mothers were mainly there to see to the supper for everyone, but they managed a dance or two also. Martha, pretty and outgoing with a bubbly personality, and being thirteen months older than Emma, was frequenting the dances in other villages too. She was a popular young lady who was asked to dance many times by different lads.

Tom taught Emma the St Bernard's Waltz and she felt so proud of her dad when he left the group of fellows with whom he was talking and walked across the floor to ask her to dance. He was a tall, good-looking man with his dark hair combed back and wearing his pin-striped suit and with his black shoes well-polished.
'Like this, Emma,' Tom instructed, as the band struck up. He was very pleased to lead this tall, slim and bonny daughter of his, to the dance floor. 'Keep in time to the music.

Sideways, one step, two, three. Then the other way, one two. Backwards two,' he continued, gently pushing Emma towards the centre of the floor. 'Out again and round you go,' swirling her round. 'Then a few waltz steps and we repeat it all.' Emma thought he danced beautifully. She picked up the steps easily although she was so tense, she felt quite wooden. 'Just relax, lass,' whispered her dad. You're doing great.' Emma never forgot that special night.

'Why didn't mam come?' she queried, as they made their way round the dance floor. Tom hesitated for a while before answering.

'She's just feeling a bit under the weather. Christmas is a busy time for her.'

'He seems a bit cagey,' Emma pondered. 'But isn't telling me. I guess they will eventually,' and with that, she put the question to the back of her mind and concentrated on the dance steps.

Much later, in the early hours of the morning, long after the dance had finished, the two sisters shared their thoughts and secrets. Firstly, Martha expressed how thrilled she'd been because halfway through the evening, the lad from High Acres sauntered across the dance floor and asked her for a dance. His fair hair was beautifully combed into waves but with a fringe hanging down to his thick, blond eyebrows, unlike most of the lads whose hair was sleeked back with brylcreem. He'd looked embarrassed when approaching her. Martha felt her face redden as she'd stood up and joined him on the dance floor.

'He's called Paul,' she'd whispered to Emma, when re-joining her, afterwards. 'He comes in the holidays or weekends to stay with his uncle on the farm. That's all I found out. He's dishy, though, isn't he?' Emma agreed. She'd only danced a couple of times, once with Uncle Jack and once with her dad, but this being her very first time, she'd soaked up the atmosphere and enjoyed watching. She didn't mention to Jack that she knew who he was, as she didn't know what to say but felt very comfortable dancing with him knowing that he was her uncle. She was determined to practise dancing at evening recreation once she returned to boarding school.

In these wee small hours, the girls discussed the knowledge of Jack Netherfield being their uncle, this being the earliest opportunity they'd had, to talk about it.

'It's weird,' whispered Martha. 'I've read about such things in women's magazines that mam buys at Whitby when she goes shopping. Fancy something like this happening in our family. It's unbelievable really.'

'I wonder why he's called Netherfield,' voiced Emma. 'If he is dad's brother, he'd be a Holmes, wouldn't he? It must be his mam's surname.'

'Or maybe his stepdad's,' suggested Martha, 'that is, if his mam married someone and changed his name. Quite intriguing, isn't it.' The girls deliberated for some time but without coming to any conclusions, before slowly drifting off to sleep.

On returning to boarding school in January, Emma was delighted to find that in the dormitory, she'd been moved again, this time to the garden side. It was much quieter that the street side as it overlooked the convent gardens and as the corridor was a dead end, there was no stream of girls

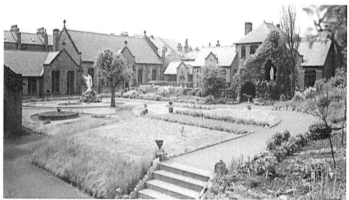

The Convent Gardens

walking past. Emma loved it. As the weeks went by, Emma was finally becoming more confident in herself and no longer as reliant as she had been, on the weekly letter from home although she loved the news from Martha who seemed to be taking over more and more from Mary in letter writing.

Martha's letters were snippets of news about boys and dances and lifts home on motor bikes.
'All very exciting stuff,' thought Emma.

Their form teacher, Miss Watson, a very enthusiastic teacher, was constantly trying to stimulate her pupils. This term she'd decided to have a Senior Choral Speaking Group and enter it into the annual competition at the Festival held in May at Whitby. Many schools in the area, participated.
'Anyone one who would like to join, can stay back on Thursday evenings and we'll practise. I'm sure there are some good speakers amongst you,' their teacher concluded, before starting the geography lesson.
'Are you going to join?' Emma asked Faith.
'I'm thinking about it.'
'Well, I'm going to,' Emma said, decisively. 'We will have to get permission, but if we stay back to practise, we'll miss the walk. I don't enjoy it much on school nights, walking in procession with a nun in tow. We might be able to go to the boarders' room and chat afterwards too, until they return, depending on how long the session takes.'

Emma had already decided to join the Senior School Choir and missed one weekday walk because of the practises. She enjoyed singing as the Holmes family spent many evenings together having a singsong. Mary, as well as playing her ukulele banjo, also joined in with the singing as she had a lovely sweet-singing voice. Tom was in the church choir and was a deep baritone singer. The children learnt many old Irish songs and ballads singing with their parents.
'Joining the Choral Speaking Group will be another way to break the routine, too,' Emma thought, delightedly. 'Two activities where I can miss the walk.' She was kicking against the rigidness of discipline and any excuse to opt out of the routine was pleasing to her.

The weekend before half-term, Emma was feeling out of sorts. She couldn't understand what was wrong with herself but was wishing she was at home. Excitement was brewing among the boarders because of the impending holiday but she struggled through the Sunday, with no appetite and little enthusiasm for anything, although she tried, when talking with Faith who was doing remarkably well this term considering she'd spent her first Christmas without her mam. Emma was hoping Faith could come to the farm with her for half-term and although Faith was waiting for a reply from her sister about this, she didn't think it would be a problem and was looking forward to visiting Bankside farm again.

'I don't know why I'm feeling like this,' she thought, dragging herself out of bed on Monday morning. 'I just want to curl up in bed and see mam and Martha and the rest of them.'

'You don't look very well,' voiced Faith, as they walked down the corridor to the hall for assembly. 'Are you feeling okay?'

'I don't feel right,' responded Emma. 'I feel like a dead weight with no energy.'

As the day proceeded, Emma was feeling worse. After evening prayers, instead of lining up to go to recreation in the big hall, Emma asked Mother Colette if she could go straight to bed.

'Whatever for?' questioned the nun.

'Please Mother. I feel ill,' replied Emma, not knowing what else to say as she didn't know what was wrong with her. Mother Colette was beginning to feel a little worried as this was the third boarder to ask her.

'I hope it's not just mollycoddling yourself, Emma. Go on then, if you must.' Emma turned away, upset at this rather curt response, so unlike Mother Colette, she thought. She made for the stairs, her eyes brimming with tears. She dragged her weary body up the flights of stairs to the dormitory feeling weak but hot and sweating. She slowly undressed, put on her pyjamas and crawled into bed full of self-pity and wishing she was at home.

The next morning, Emma struggled out of bed, feeling dreadful. When she unbuttoned her pyjama top, she saw them. Little pink spots! She pulled on her dressing gown and wandered around to the centre of the dormitory to see Mother Teresa and tell her.

'Yes, Emma?'

'Look, I've got spots and I don't feel very well,' Emma said, opening her pyjama top, a little. Mother Teresa glanced at the few spots.

'Don't be silly. They're nothing. But go back to bed if you

must.' Sadly, Emma went back to her cubicle and crawled under the blankets.

'No sympathy and understanding, here, then,' she thought, disconsolately, 'like I would have got at home.' Her eyes filled up and a few silent few tears trickled down her cheeks onto her pillow. She tried to go to sleep but was tossing and turning, being very restless and hot, before finally nodding off. Meanwhile, despite her rather brusque response to Emma, Mother Teresa felt concerned enough to report it.

About an hour later, Emma was awakened by the tall, kindly head nun, Mother Margaret.

'Let me see, Emma,' she stated gently. 'You're running a temperature. Yes, those are spots. We will call a doctor to look at you. Stay in bed. I will ask Mother Teresa to bring you a little something to eat and a drink.' As this nun was quite motherly towards her, Emma felt reassured but wanted to cry even more. Sometime later, the doctor visited along with Mother Margaret.

'Your hunch was right,' he said to the nun. 'It is German measles. If you have a spare bedroom, I'd move her. Otherwise you might have a lot more patients on your hands if they decide to visit her in here.' Mother Margaret nodded.

'Thank you, doctor. I will do that.' The doctor moved out of the cubicle followed by the nun. Emma snuggled back under the bed clothes, relieved that at least they'd know that she was genuinely ill.

Later, Emma was moved to a large empty bedroom, next door to the junior dormitory and within two days, three more girls joined her. Audrey was among them. She explained to Emma that Mother Colette had sent the rest of the boarders home early before half-term as she didn't want an epidemic on her hands.

'Well, that's what I've been told,' she said. 'We'll be here for half-term.' Emma's heart sank as she was looking forward immensely to going home and with Faith joining her. It seemed quite a while since Christmas.

'Poor Faith,' she thought, sorrowfully. 'She'll be so disappointed.'

'Good morning, ladies. And how are our patients today?'

Mother Colette sounded very cheerful. 'Letters for you two,' she said, walking across to the two girls in the far beds, 'and a parcel for you, Audrey.' She looked at Emma. 'I think you are ready to get up today for an hour or so.' Emma nodded. 'Your father telephoned. Apparently, the bus route from Whitby is blocked by snow. He was going to tell you to take the train from Whitby to Shepton and he was to meet you there with the tractor. I told him that you won't be home for half-term. He sends his love. Faith told me that she'd been invited, but she has gone home to see her sister.' Emma bit her bottom lip to stop herself from crying, suddenly feeling very homesick especially at the mention of her dad, the tractor and the snow. Disappointment was etched on her face.

Audrey was tearing off the brown paper from her parcel. Inside she took out a selection of sweets, fruit, a magazine, pink writing paper and envelopes and a get-well card. The other girls watched. Emma was envious. She knew Mary was busy at home and it was difficult to go shopping at a moment's notice. Emma wasn't expecting anything. Martha told her in her last letter that their mam was preoccupied, but that she didn't know why. Audrey very kindly shared her sweets and fruit with the three girls and Emma enjoyed the goodies. Later in the morning, she dressed and wandered down to the boarders' room. It was unoccupied and not at all homely.
'I'll write to Martin,' Emma thought. 'Then, maybe, he'll write back if he knows I've missed going home.'

It was a strange half-term for Emma, with no walks or orderly lining up or night prayers or supervised recreation. Only the four of them, when the other girls recovered, sitting together for meals. The nuns left them on their own most of the time, to do as they wished, but checked that they were going to bed at the correct time. Luckily for Emma, Audrey was able to lend her books and teenage magazines.
'You'll enjoy the *Dear Aunt Sally* question page, Emma. It's all about boyfriends and relationships. Did you know that someone can have an operation to change sex? I read about it in a magazine at home.' Emma shook her head. She'd never heard of anything like that. 'I've read about

parents having affairs and children with different fathers,' Audrey continued, trying to impress Emma with her worldly knowledge of grown-up stuff.

'Audrey knows so much,' Emma thought. 'How can anyone change their sex,' she wondered, thinking it must be a wild exaggeration. 'Thanks for these, Audrey. It will help to pass the time,' she replied, taking the books and magazines. 'I'll let you have them back when I've finished with them. I love reading,' she added, appreciating Audrey's kindness. As Emma was glancing through the magazine, she began thinking about her grandad and Uncle Jack. 'Maybe there will be a story in the magazine like that,' she mused.

Eventually, a letter arrived from Mary telling Emma how disappointed they'd all been about her not coming home. *Ask if I can come and take you out one Saturday to make up for missing the holiday*, she wrote. *Mrs Williams says she will come with me and we'll do a bit of shopping together.* Emma was delighted and approached the nun after evening prayers, but Mother Colette wasn't enthusiastic about this request. She wasn't keen on boarders being allowed out on Saturdays as she thought it might unsettle them during school term and she felt for those to whom this would never happen because of their home life. She reluctantly gave her permission because boarders, at their first interview, were told that this would be allowed.

Arrangements were made. Emma wondered if Martha might come but on arriving, her mother explained that Martha was needed at home to mind the younger children. It was a great effort for Mary as the journey alone was well over an hour and walking to the convent for Emma, added time to the journey, but Mary was enjoying the freedom of a day out without children. Emma followed behind her mother and Mrs Williams as they nattered away, walking down Queen Street. On listening to them, she realised just how broad their Yorkshire accents were, sounding totally out of place in Scarborough. Her feelings were mixed.

'I seem to be moving into a different culture, not kind of belonging in quite the same way,' Emma thought. 'It's strange.'

She followed them into shop after shop until Mary stopped, realising that she was so immersed in looking around these fascinating stores and enjoying this special time that she wasn't paying much attention to her daughter.
'Is there anything you particularly need, Emma? You're getting so tall.' Emma shook her head. 'Let's go and have a bite and a cup of tea, then. It's lovely seeing you. You can tell us about school while we sit.'

'You needn't see me back, Mam,' said Emma, later in the afternoon when Mary said it was time to get home. 'You might as well go straight to the bus stop as I know my way.' She hugged her mother. 'Give Amy and Jacob a hug from me. Tell Martha I love her letters. I'll see you all soon, at Easter.' She watched them go off in the direction of the bus station and made her way back to the convent, deep in thought about her family and her school.

Emma's feelings of being different, re-surfaced when back at home for the Easter holidays especially when she wore her

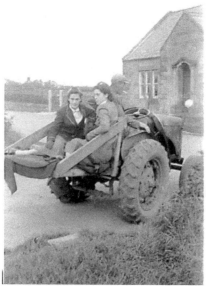

Emma (left) and Martha in link-box, leaving Windrush after church

brown school blazer for church. Her school coat was discarded as she'd outgrown it and at present, she didn't possess one. She loved wearing the blazer. It was smart with fawn and brown braiding around the edges and displaying the school badge on the pocket. The blazers were designed originally without braiding and only recently were available with braiding, for the youngest pupils. Older girls were asked to buy and sew braiding onto their blazers. Emma didn't have a one the first year and when finally obtaining one, was told by Mary to buy it on the large size, as she was growing all the time. She painstakingly sewed the braiding on. She felt very smart when first wearing it to go to church in Windrush but then began to feel out of place and a little estranged from her local peer group whom she bumped into.

'It seems to me,' she thought, 'that I don't feel like I belong with my peers at school and yet, I feel different to the people at home. It's like being in no-man's land. I don't fit in anywhere.'

'Dad says you have something to tell me, Mam,' stated Emma, one morning towards the end of the Easter break, whilst laying the table for breakfast. She'd been to the cowshed with a mug of tea for Tom and he'd informed her that Mary had some news for her but wanted to wait until Faith went home. Faith, who'd spent most of the two weeks with them, left the previous day for Bartown to see her sister Rose and her uncles before returning to school.

'Ask her when you go in. Little ones don't know yet,' Tom added, cautiously. 'Keep it to yourself for now.' Emma was curious. Her mam was much brighter than at Christmas and seemed well. The older children were out with Tom, including Mark, who was feeding the hens. Amy was sitting on the clip mat crossed-legged, making a garage with wooden stacking bricks with Jacob. Mary smiled.

'I thought you would have noticed.'

Emma looked at her mother and gave this some thought. Mary moved closer and whispered, 'I'm having another baby, but we're not telling the younger children yet.' Emma looked surprised and then smiled, as this news sunk in. She didn't quite know what to say. 'I've bought you some wool,' her mam continued. 'You can knit a matinee coat for the baby, with bootees and hat to match, if you like when you go back. I have some old patterns and we have plenty of knitting needles.'

'I'd love to,' replied Emma, excitedly, now she'd absorbed this information. 'Wait till I tell Faith.' She paused. 'Does that mean that Faith can't come to stay in summer?'

'The baby's due at the beginning of August. Maybe she could come towards the end of the holidays. I'll see how I feel. She could possibly come the next half-term though, if you like.'

'What are you knitting?' asked Audrey on the second evening of the summer term, noticing Emma using thin white wool whilst reading instructions from a baby clothes pattern laying on the table. 'Somebody having a baby?' Emma paused before answering as she remembered Tom telling her to keep it quiet. She wondered for a minute if she should tell Audrey but thinking that it probably didn't matter as Mary would be telling the children soon. Who could Audrey disclose the information to, anyway, she concluded.

'My mam is expecting again,' Emma replied, feeling slightly embarrassed but not knowing why.'

'Another baby!' exclaimed Audrey.

'Well, I think it's lovely,' said Faith, coming up behind Audrey. Emma had secretly told Faith, on arriving back at boarding school, as she trusted her friend to keep it quiet. Now the news was out but she didn't think it a problem. Audrey changed the conversation by relating her exploits over the holidays and nothing more was said to Emma about the expected baby. Whenever she had a spare moment after finishing her homework, out came the knitting. It was a lacy pattern and quite complicated, but Emma was able to concentrate in the silence of the boarders' room and was hoping to finish the garments before the end of term.

'They are so cute,' Faith commented. 'You're very talented. I can't knit a stitch.'

'My mam knits loads,' replied Emma. 'I've been knitting for years.'

As soon as the pupils returned to school, the Choral Speaking Group increased its weekly practise, as the date of

the competition at the Whitby Festival, was fast approaching. 'I wish you were coming,' Emma said to Faith. 'I love the poem we're doing. It's *The Brook* by Alfred, Lord Tennyson. It has thirteen verses and reciting it, reminds me of Bankside especially the first line of the third verse: *Till last by Philip's farm I flow*, as I think of us paddling in the beck at the bottom of our pasture at Bankside, knowing the water flowed on, eventually joining the river Esk.'
'I left it too late to take part, but I hope you win,' Faith responded, encouragingly.

'Make sure you are wearing your uniform,' stated Miss Watson, at the end of classes, the day before the big event. We will make the journey by bus. Be prepared for a lengthy day as there are lots of competitions with many schools participating. Bring packed lunches and we'll hope for good weather so that we can sit on the sea front to eat.' It was an exciting day, thoroughly enjoyed by the girls who also managed to schedule, in their busy day, a walk up the ninety-nine steps to the Abbey ruins. The views out to sea were spectacular with the sun glistening across the waters. The icing on the cake was that they came first in their category and their teachers were delighted.

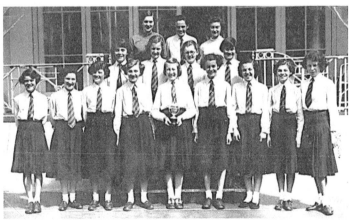

Cup-winning Choral Speaking Group

A photograph was taken of the two teachers accompanying them, along with the fourteen pupils participating and with one lucky girl holding the winners' cup. The only embarrassing moment for Emma was when Miss Watson called her to stand between the teachers for the photograph, but she daren't refuse. 'Mother Colette will be pleased,' enthused Miss Watson, after the picture was taken. 'Well done, everyone.' Emma was sorry that it was over as she wouldn't have an excuse to miss the walk on Thursdays, but they could go swimming instead, she thought.

Apart from swimming, there were other highlights in the summer term. In the convent grounds, there were tennis courts and as recreation after supper was outside, weather permitting, the tennis courts were soon taken up. Girls sat on benches chatting and one or two occupied themselves bashing a tennis ball against the high stone wall at one end of the recreation space. Maria and Emma spent many enjoyable evenings practising their strokes. It was a shame, Emma thought, that they still went to bed at eight thirty on these light nights.
'I can read in bed till much later,' she mused, trying to look on the bright side.

'Faith,' called Emma as she caught up with her friend, after classes, one afternoon. 'Martha has written. You can come at half-term, if you like. Mam told her to tell me. It's only Friday to Tuesday but we might be able to go to a dance.' Faith's eyes lit up.
'That's great. I'll tell Rose next time I write. It doesn't matter about a dance. Just coming will be lovely.'
'You haven't met Uncle Jack yet, either, have you. It's an interesting story.' Emma proceeded to tell Faith the background. 'He's kind and gives us lifts sometimes to church or Whitby to shop. He doesn't tend to go to dances much unless dad is going. You're used to uncles though, aren't you?' Faith nodded.

The girls spent an enjoyable four days at Bankside. Martha was staying over at a girlfriend's house on the Saturday night whilst Emma and Faith stayed in and played cards with Tom and Tim, instead of going dancing. Faith didn't meet Uncle Jack but thoroughly enjoyed her stay. She secretly thought that Tim was a very handsome lad and playing cards with him was all part of the fun. His hazel eyes twinkled when he smiled at her. She loved the Holmes family.

It was a week or two after half-term that Emma began having problems with her shoes as she realised that they were wearing out. Eventually a small hole appeared in the sole of one and it gradually got bigger. Emma was confiding in Maria about this, one morning, as they were making their way early to Mass in the chapel.

'It's happened to me before,' Maria replied, on listening to Emma's tale of woe. 'I cut out a foot shape from thick card and put it inside my shoe. It worked, but you may have to change the card as it will wear out quickly.' Emma thought this great advice. The next time a boarder received a parcel in a shoe box, she asked for the empty box and after flattening it, put it in her locker. The following morning, because she'd been to early morning Mass, she found time in the boarders' room, whilst the other boarders were making their beds, to take the flattened card, measure her foot on it, cut out a shape and place it inside her shoe.

'Perfect,' she thought, as it was quite a strong shoe box. She was delighted to have dealt with her dilemma.

When writing her customary letter home, the following Saturday, Emma explained to her parents the situation about her shoe and how she'd rectified the problem. Almost a week later, a parcel arrived for her.

'Most unusual,' she thought, unknotting the string. Ripping off the paper she could see it was a shoe box and inside were a pair of shoes, size seven, quite smart with a small block heel and light brown in colour. Mary had enclosed a little note to say that the shoes were an early birthday present for her fourteenth birthday at the end of July. Although Emma appreciated how thoughtful and generous it was of her parents, she hadn't the heart to tell them, when writing her next letter home, that heels weren't suitable for everyday use at school. 'I'll tell them I've worn the shoes,' she thought, 'which I have, once, but I won't mention that they're a bit big and slip up and down when I walk. I'll explain when I see them. It was kind of them, though. At least I've more card now to hopefully keep me going till the end of term. I'll need it with the other shoe staring to wear through,' she mused.

It seemed to Emma that everything was wearing out. After almost three years at boarding school, her uniform brown skirt, as well as looking decidedly short, was also showing signs of wear. An area at the back of it was becoming shiny and was beginning to look somewhat threadbare. 'I could darn it very neatly with brown cotton,' she thought. She asked around and eventually borrowed a reel and painstakingly, one evening in her cubicle, threaded the cotton up and down the thin part at the back.
'Not bad, that,' she told herself. 'You can hardly tell I've darned it.' She was pleased with her efforts but was glad that end of term was approaching.

Emma still did not have any colouring pencils but most of the time she managed without them. When it was essential to colour something, she borrowed from one of the other girls. She'd never mentioned this to her parents as it seemed of minor importance. Rita, who worked alongside Emma, since joining the form when the two parallel forms had been remixed after the first year at school, had lots of colouring pencils. In lessons, when using a different colour was helpful, and knowing Emma's predicament, Rita lent Emma hers. Occasionally this happened in a maths lesson something which had not gone unnoticed by Miss Markey, their maths teacher.

Rumours had been going around for weeks about Miss Markey possibly retiring at the end of term and on finishing her lesson the following week, she finally confirmed this with her pupils. A day or two before the end of term when she was saying her goodbyes, as the girls filed out for lunch, she beckoned Rita and Emma to stand aside.
'My two, star pupils,' she said, after the other girls left. 'A little gift for each of you. You've worked hard and given me no trouble.' The girls thanked her and took their presents with them.

Emma opened hers discreetly, when walking down the corridor to the dining hall. It was a box of colouring pencils.

'That's so kind of her,' Emma thought. 'How understanding and thoughtful.' She was delighted and made a quick dash back to her form room to put them in her desk. 'I'll be able to use them in my other lessons too, next term,' she thought. She felt very joyful as she made her way to the refectory.
'I'll write,' was Emma's parting shot to Faith as the girls went their separate ways on the last day of term. 'Maybe later in August, you might be able to come. I'll see how things are.' Faith nodded. She wasn't looking forward to the long summer break. She missed her mam and going to the pictures wasn't quite the same without her. At times like these, Faith ached for her.
'It would be great to get a letter, Emma. I'm really going to miss being with you all. Let me know when the baby arrives.'
'I'll do that. I'm sorry you can't come,' her friend replied.
They parted, both feeling a little sad.

'I'm so glad to see you,' Mary greeted her when Emma walked into the farmhouse kitchen, followed by Tom who had met her at the bus stop. Emma looked at Mary. Her mother was very heavily pregnant and was struggling with her family and housework and was looking forward to Emma helping her. Emma thought her mother's belly was enormous but didn't like to comment. She kept glancing at it. She's forgotten how big a pregnant woman can look.
'Aye, she'll be a good help to you, Mary,' stated Tom, placing Emma's case on the cement floor. 'I'll get back to work now. Get changed and give your mam a hand, will you.' He walked out and Emma sighed.
'So, this is what's it's going to be like', she thought. 'Never mind, things will be better when mam has the baby,' she reckoned, hopefully.

Mary had paddled around in great discomfort in the last few weeks of pregnancy, feeling very weary. She was glad to hand the reigns over to Emma, now fourteen and growing up. Martha, having celebrated her fifteenth birthday at the end of June, left school for good in the July. She worked full-time at home, mainly outside on the farm helping Tom but more recently inside to assist Mary. Tim also finished at the grammar school this summer as he'd celebrated his sixteenth birthday in April. He'd found part-time work on one of the farms locally and although looking for more hours, was able to give a hand to his dad. With Emma home to oversee the household, Martha returned to working outside with Tom, much to the envy of her sister, now engaged with cooking and cleaning and sorting out the younger siblings. 'School holidays are not really holidaying,' she surmised. 'Just a different way of living.'

The baby sister was born at the beginning of August, days after the holidays began. Mary originally planned to go into a nursing home at Whitby to give birth but changed her mind. She'd already given birth six times at home and at the last minute decided she couldn't face leaving Tom and the children. Emma was glad that the baby had arrived so soon after they'd broken up from school, as she was still hoping that Faith might be allowed to come later in the holidays. 'Maybe Uncle Jack would take them to a dance as Faith hadn't yet been to one of the village dances,' she thought. Martha went dancing regularly at Shepton, a village a few miles away, where there was one held in the village hall each Saturday evening. Emma thought it would be fun to join her as Martha knew lads with motor bikes and sometimes came home on one.

There was a lot of commotion on the day that Mary went into labour. Her labour pains began in the early hours of the morning and it was shortly after Tom had been to Windrush to telephone for help, that the midwife arrived.
'I can hear mam shouting a bit,' whispered Emma to Martha, who'd come in to help her with the little ones and getting breakfast ready, on Tom's instructions. They stood together outside the sitting room where the midwife was attending to Mary. Earlier, Emma helped prepare the bed on her mother's instructions by putting layers of old newspaper under a worn sheet that was covering a piece of rubber sheeting. Mary's shouts and groans were increasing in volume. As Tom walked into the back kitchen, he heard her and rushed into the bedroom. Martha and Emma scuttled back into the kitchen where Jacob and Amy seemed oblivious to what was going on. They were happily absorbed with their crayons and colouring books. Mark was out with Tim. Then there was a baby's cry and the girls gazed at

each other.

'It's come,' Martha whispered. 'I wonder what it is.' They waited. Eventually the sitting room door opened. Tom came out, smiling.

'You've got a baby sister,' he told them. 'The midwife wasn't too pleased with me going in, in my mucky working clothes, but I was there for Mary. Your mam's okay now. See to breakfast for us, will you, lasses. You can make a cup of tea for the midwife and your mam. They'll be ready for one, shortly. Make sure the bairns are fed. I just need to warm up the water to wash the new one with.' He took the kettle through and the girls heard him speak to the midwife. Returning to the kitchen, he placed a large ball of wrapped up newspaper on the fire to burn, before going outside to finish in the cowshed. Emma and Martha eyed the burning paper. Blood was seeping out of it as the flames licked around it.

'It's like when a cow calves, I suppose,' commented Martha. 'You know, Emma. All that water and blood and stuff that comes out. Poor mam. We'd better get them that cup of tea. Mam might like a slice of bread and butter.' The girls were rather subdued as they busied themselves.

The midwife came out and smiled at the little family.

'You can go in and see your new little sister,' she said, 'but your mam is tired. Don't stay long. Take that little lad's hand and keep hold of him. I'll have my cup of tea in here,' she said, noticing the tea and buttered bread on the tray. Martha reached out to Jacob.

'Come here, Jacob. We can see mam. She's in bed.' After removing a cup for the midwife, Emma picked up the tray and told Amy to follow her. They trooped into the bedroom and gazed at the tiny baby in Mary's arms. The baby was snuggled up in a blanket, but they could see that she had lots of black hair and big brown eyes. Her face was smooth with little pink lips. She was looking around.

'She's beautiful, isn't she,' said Emma, almost in a whisper. Mary smiled.

'You can kiss her,' she invited, 'on her forehead,' she added, holding the little mite out. The children took turns, each planting a gentle kiss on their tiny baby sister's face, before leaving the room. Emma was last to leave after placing the tray at the side of the bed. She thought that her mam looked very tired.

Baby Miriam cried quite a lot at first and was always feeding. She seemed to take up all of Mary's wakening hours. There was an abundance of washing for the girls to see to. Both a muslin and a terry nappy were used each time that the baby was changed. The soiled muslin ones were cleaned off before being soaked in a bucket of water along with the wet terry ones. These added to the numerous items of clothing constantly piling up from the rest of the family. Tom lit the tiny fire under the copper boiler in the back kitchen, almost daily, for the nappies to be washed in very hot water. Other clothes were washed in the hand-driven washing machine. It was hard work. Mrs Williams from the neighbouring farm, came a couple of times at first, making sure Mary stayed in bed, resting and sleeping.

Emma and Martha looked after everything as best they could, including the washing and baking. They also looked after their younger siblings with Tom calling in, as and when he could, checking on his wife and making sure that the children were okay.
'It's a good job it's holiday time,' commented Martha, one morning, as she was washing the pots in the bowl on the kitchen table and putting them on the tray to drip. Emma was drying and putting away.
'At least, there are two of us.' Emma added. 'I'm going to write to Faith. There's no way she can come these holidays with all that's going on. She's going to be disappointed.'

Eventually, Mary slowly took over, wearily plodding through the routine whilst longing for sleep.
'Having a baby in summer is a bonus, as the clothes dry quickly in the orchard,' she thought, one bright, sunny morning. She was pegging out the nappies and remembering the dreary, damp weather in the November following Jacob's birth. She was trying to think positively. Many times, Mary told the children to go out and play whilst she dozed in the rocking chair, often with the baby asleep across her lap. Work continued inside the house and out in the fields.

One Friday afternoon, whilst the little ones were happily playing, the two older girls went upstairs to see if they could empty one of the drawers of the old, dark chest, where everyone's clothes were kept. There wasn't enough room in the chest for all the clothes and many were left in piles at the end of the beds. Martha and Emma decided they'd take out their clothes from the chest to make more room. Then by emptying one drawer completely into the others, they would have an empty drawer just for themselves. They were happily sorting clothes when Mary shouted from the sitting room. They'd disturbed her sleeping by their chatter and noise. She told her daughters to leave it and she'd sort it out later. Miriam was crotchety and Mary wasn't coping well and feeling dejected because she couldn't satisfy her baby with her own milk. It was inevitable that Miriam would need a bottle feed, much to Mary's disappointment.

'Never mind,' said Martha to Emma. 'Mam's always tired now. Maybe she'll feel better when Miriam sleeps more. We'll be able to take a turn at giving the baby a bottle and that might help. There's another dance at Shepton tomorrow night. We'll enjoy that.' The girls loved the dances. Emma, having celebrated her fourteenth birthday at the end of July, was now allowed to go regularly with Martha in the holidays. Martha gave Emma a cigarette sometimes too, when they joined in with some of the lads smoking.

'As long as you're up next morning,' instructed Tom. They found the dances great fun.

'How will we get tomorrow night,' Emma asked her sister, later in the evening. 'Have you made plans again?'
'I thought we'd walk this time, across the valley and up the other side. There is a sheep track through the heather which we'll pick up. It leads across the top moor and then we'll walk down the other side and join the tarmac road into Shepton. We needn't worry about getting back home as there are lads with motor bikes who will give us a ride, or we'll squeeze into someone's car or join others in sharing a taxi. There's a farmer who runs one and is used to a gang of us piling in.'
'That sounds great,' Emma replied, looking forward to the following evening. She was wondering if that lad who worked at Uncle Jack's, would be there. Martha had seen him a

couple of times when she'd visited with her dad. The girls were curious about him. He didn't turn up and neither did Paul from High Acres, but there were other lads who asked Emma for a dance and Martha was constantly being partnered. The girls arrived safely home after a hilarious ride, sitting on each other's laps, as there were so many squeezed into the taxi.

On rare occasions, Emma helped outside with Martha. At these times, Martha told her younger sister about the lads she liked and that one or two had kissed her.
'Just be warned,' she advised. Emma loved being outside with her dad. He was treating them older and let them light woodbines for him. He gave Martha one sometimes and she shared it with Emma. It didn't taste too good at first, but Emma, thinking it was part of growing up, persevered and began to enjoy a little smoke. It was a different world to the one she experienced at the boarding school with its discipline and routine, but back she had to go.
'But I will see Faith and the others and have a good chat. Audrey may have more books and magazines for me to read. In some ways, it's more comfortable at the convent, especially being able to have a bath,' she thought. 'It's like two different worlds I live in. I now have to go back to the other one.'

Autumn to Summer 1955

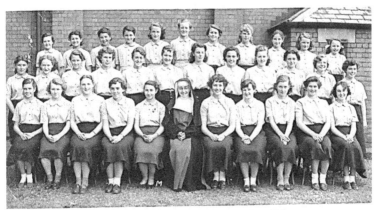

Mother Colette with Boarders 1954/55

'How was your holiday?' Emma asked Faith, on meeting up
at recreation. Faith pulled a face.
'It was a bit boring. Not half as much fun as yours, I bet.
How's the new baby?' Now Emma grimaced.
'She's lovely but cries a lot and I'd forgotten how demanding
new babies are. Me and Martha worked hard trying to keep
on top of things as mam was always tired. We did get to a
few dances though. Faith listened enviously whilst Emma
related the details. She wouldn't have minded the work. She
loved Bankside farm.

Emma was looking forward to this term because she would
have less subjects to study, leaving a possible few free
periods instead of a full timetable. On arriving at her form
room on the first morning, Emma was thinking about this,
remembering last's term's discussion with her teachers
about which options to take for her 'O' level exams held in
upper fifth year.
'Great,' she thought. 'No more History, Scripture or Art this
term.' She'd opted for Geography instead of History and as
she was obliged to take the Catholic Religious Education
exam as an additional to the listed subjects on offer, she'd
decided to drop Scripture and she'd never being much good
at drawing.

The girls were hanging around, whilst waiting for their form teacher. Unexpectedly, Mother Colette walked in. There was a quick scuffle as the girls made for their desks.
'Good morning, girls. I hope that you have come back refreshed from your summer holidays. As you know, you have an important year ahead in preparation for your chosen 'O' level exams.' She looked around at the listening girls. 'We are introducing Spanish into the school curriculum this year as a subject to be taken at 'O' level. I'll read out the names of the five pupils whom I've chosen from amongst you to take the subject.' After stating the names, Mother Colette continued, speaking directly to the girls in question. 'I know it is only two years to your exams, but I think you are capable of taking another language.' Then she addressed each one in turn, including Emma, one of the named five. 'Emma, you will need to drop Domestic Science. I've re-arranged your timetable.' When she'd finally finished speaking, she turned and greeted Miss Watson, who'd quietly walked in and was standing, waiting patiently. After the head mistress left, Miss Watson spent a couple of minutes discussing these changes with the five girls, before commencing her lesson.

Emma didn't mind dropping Domestic Science. She felt she could cook reasonably well, but taking Spanish was a surprise as she was already studying French and Latin. She hoped it was the same teacher for French who'd taught them last year as she was patient and encouraging. The previous year they'd had a different teacher and although okay generally, she was a bit sarcastic over Emma's lack of general knowledge, as happened in one of the lessons when they'd been talking about different universities.
'What do you mean, you've never heard of Eton. Everyone knows of Eton.' Emma didn't.

On another occasion, each pupil was asked to describe, in French, something about the town or place they lived in. Emma knew she couldn't describe Moorbeck, the valley where the farm was situated. She tried to describe Windrush with its two churches, two schools, one shop and a pub but she didn't know the French translation for pub. She remembered there was a bacon factory, but it was very small, she thought. She decided not to mention it as she realised that she knew next to nothing about it.

'Is that all?' the teacher questioned. Emma nodded and sat down. Most of the girls lived in Scarborough and those who spoke, had plenty to talk about, although some, like Emma, found it difficult to remember the French translations. On another occasion, they'd been asked to describe their family, but she was the only one who's dad was a farmer. She struggled with feeling she was different. She quickly looked at her timetable and was little disappointed to find that it was this teacher and not only for French, but also for Spanish. Feeling disappointed, she also noticed that she'd lost some free periods with the change of subjects.

'It's going to be a tough year,' she decided.

A few days later, as Emma was placing her books on her desk, Brenda walked up the aisle.

'Is that nicotine on your finger?' she asked. 'I spotted it yesterday.' Emma looked at her finger and realised the stain was quite noticeable.

'Actually, it must be staining from the dye that I've been using. My mam bought me some sandals in summer that were a bit light and I've been dyeing them so that I can wear them at school.' That was true, as Mary bought the dye along with the sandals and Emma wore them as indoor shoes replacing her worn-out old ones. They still weren't quite the correct colour but an improvement after dyeing. Emma wasn't unduly bothered. One of her mam's expressions was *It's a case of make-do and mend*, or in this case, dye them, she thought. The dyeing was a cover-up story though, as the stain was nicotine, but she didn't want to admit to her peer group that she smoked. Brenda wasn't convinced with the explanation and raised her eyebrows at Emma although she said no more.

A couple of weeks later when curled up in bed reading a letter from her sister, Emma was thinking about dancing and smoking and motor bikes. She remembered Brenda's comment.

'I must be more careful and not smoke the cigarettes right to the end,' she surmised. She continued reading the letter. 'She seems to have a lot of fun,' she thought, 'but maybe she just tells me the best bits.' Instead of Mary writing, Martha wrote a letter almost weekly and had being doing so for weeks in the previous term, always telling Emma of her social life and exploits with the local lads. Mary usually added a few lines at the end of Martha's letters which pleased Emma. She explained that she was now so busy with baby Miriam and missing her little helper, as she called Emma, that she didn't have time to write, but that she knew her daughter would understand. 'I suppose mam thinks that I enjoy Martha's news and I do, but I still like to hear from my mam,' she thought, pensively, folding up the letter and putting it in her locker, before settling down to sleep.

Now into her lower fifth year, Emma was quite accustomed to boarding school and was confident within herself, but there were still incidents cropping up in school hours that were a challenge for her. One such occurrence was in an English lesson, even though she enjoyed the subject. The English teacher was new to this set of pupils, as they'd had a different one in the previous years. Miss Kirkham was tall, slim and elegant, with her short brown hair stylishly cut and she usually wore black high heeled shoes, giving her more height. She sometimes wore her black, long graduation gown, looking very impressive.

The problem in the lesson early on in term, was when this teacher gave some of the pupils, including Emma, a speaking part as they were studying a Shakespearean play. Emma did not like doing this as they each had to stand up when speaking their character part. At a later English lesson, the teacher did not choose her, but called her to one side at the end of it. Out of ear shot of the other pupils, she spoke to her.
'Emma, although you are clever at English, I noticed in the previous lesson when I asked you to read that you were uncomfortable with it. You seemed embarrassed and I gather you do not like being in the spotlight. I chose other pupils today and, in the future, to prevent any anxiety, I won't ask you again. It will not affect your understanding of the subject and your written work is good.' Emma already thought this teacher excellent at her subject and one of the best teachers they'd had.

'Thank you,' she replied. 'What a great teacher,' she thought.' One less worry.' She was so grateful to her.

There were lighter moments during this heavy term of studying especially when playing netball or hockey. Emma looked forward to these lessons as a time of freedom outdoors but realised, since becoming much taller, just how short her shorts were, on her long legs. When Mary purchased the obligatory school uniform shorts for PE, she allowed for growth. The shorts were of a thick dark brown material and heavily flared.
'They were down to my knees in my first year,' mused Emma, one afternoon when changing for hockey. 'I know mam wanted them to last, but they're heading towards my thighs now. I'm not sure if they'll still be respectable next year if I keep growing.' She wasn't the only one with this dilemma. 'Are your shorts shrinking?' she cheekily asked Rita, looking at her healthy display of upper legs.' Audrey chipped in.
'At least we're all in the same boat with our very short shorts.' They laughed.

The girls made their way to the hockey field outside the convent grounds. Hockey was an additional sport taught by Miss Watson; the girls having played netball from arriving in first year. Emma played the right back position and was very energetic flying around the field with her hockey stick. That was, until a break in the game, when she was larking about with another player and split her tongue caused by a collision with a very hard stick.
'What's the matter with you?' Miss Watson asked, as she joined the huddle of girls around Emma.
'I've accidently cut my tongue.'
'Show me.' Emma put out her tongue, revealing a bright red open gash. 'It will heal but I can't imagine how you managed to collide with a hockey stick,' was her comment before blowing her whistle to recommence the game. 'You'd better sit out this half.' Emma sighed. She loved her game of hockey.
'It's almost as much fun as netball,' she thought, dejectedly, having to sit on the bench and watch. That evening, Emma ate gingerly, as her tongue was very sore. It was days

before eating became comfortable.

'There always seems to be problems,' Emma thought, one morning, struggling with so many text and exercise books when taking them from her locker in the boarders' room. Throughout her school years since starting, she'd carried her books around as she didn't possess a satchel. 'I really could do with a satchel. We seem to have so many books this year. I guess it's because of our 'O' levels next year.' It was well into the term and homework was increasing. With her arms full of books and holding her pens in her hand, Emma made her way down the stairs and along the corridors to the main hall. No-one was allowed into their form room until after assembly. There was a lot of jostling in the hall as the day girls milled around chatting.

Eventually, Mother Colette walked onto the stage and clapped her hands. The talking ceased and the girls shuffled into their rows for morning prayers. Emma placed her pile of books on the floor with her pens on top. Prayers began. Suddenly there was a commotion in the next row of girls, adjacent to Emma. One of the pupils was having an epileptic fit and lay sprawled out on the floor, her arms and legs thrashing. Pupils moved aside and others were trying to help. Emma's books were knocked over and scattered amidst the chaos. Along with some girls who were scrambling to help, she hastily retrieved her belongings with a quick thankyou to those handing back her books.

Mother Colette clapped her hands and dismissed everyone, whilst a couple of teachers, having rushed over from the stage, were giving assistance to the pupil on the floor. Emma, carrying her books, left the hall, a little embarrassed but hiding her emotions as best she could. On arriving in her form room, she went to her desk, but no-one commented on the situation as their teacher was already present and they knuckled down to pay attention. Emma was feeling subdued, firstly, as she was quite shaken about the girl who'd taken ill, not having witnessed anything like that before, and secondly, about not having a satchel.

'I guess I'll have to manage without one,' she thought, resignedly.

Half-term was soon upon them.

'You can come, you know,' Emma told Faith. 'Miriam is sleeping through the night now and my mam is feeling a lot better.'

'That's good. I'll tell Rose in my next letter.' Faith was delighted.

During half-term, Mary showed Emma her new coat, as her second-hand school uniform coat, too big three years ago when she started the grammar school, no longer fit her. She'd been wearing her school blazer throughout the summer term and up to half -term this school year. Mary, noticing that Emma was quite tall for a fourteen-year-old, commented how Emma had 'shot up,' when home in the summer holidays.

'It was in a sale,' her mother explained. 'I knew you'd need a coat, now it's autumn and the weather's getting cooler. I know the colour is a little lighter in shade than the uniform brown, but it was such a bargain. I thought it would be okay for you.' Her daughter tried on the coat. It had padded shoulders and a broad belt and a pleat up the back which swung out when Emma twirled around. 'What do you think, Faith?' questioned Mary, noticing Faith's serious expression. Faith pondered, unsure of how to answer.

'It is a bit different from the brown uniform coats, but I think it will be okay,' she said, not wanting to upset Mary or Emma.

'And I guess you girls will be going dancing tomorrow night,' said Mary, changing the subject, on realising that the coat had not gone down too well. 'Jack may take you, he said, if you can find your way home.'

'Mam, that's great. Faith, you'll finally meet Uncle Jack.'

At half eight the following evening, Jack Netherfield arrived and the three girls, as Martha was going too, walked out to his van, after Emma introduced Faith.

'At last we meet,' Jack said, opening the back door of the van. 'I've heard plenty about you.' Faith smiled.

'So have I about you.'

'I hope it was favourable.'

'Oh, it was,' she declared, happily, before joining Emma in the back of the van. Martha was sitting up front with Jack. After dropping the girls at the dance hall, Jack Netherfield parked up outside the village pub and on entering, ordered a pint and settled himself in a quiet corner. He was thinking about Faith. She seemed a very pleasant girl, he thought, from the short time he'd met her, but something about her was stirring at the back of his mind and he couldn't quite name it.

'Now, Jack,' called out one of the locals, wandering over to him. With that, Jack, put aside his thoughts for a later time.

It was after half-term that the question of suitability of Emma's coat re-surfaced.

'Come on, Flash Harry,' Emma heard the voice calling when putting on her outdoor shoes for the customary walk. She grinned. This was her latest nickname with reference to her outdoor coat. The boarders had watched *The Girls of St Trinians* in the boarders' room with the nuns, as a special treat, one Sunday evening just before the school broke up for half-term. Flash Harry was quite a character in the film, tall and slim and identified by his long brown raincoat with padded shoulders and a broad belt, not unlike the coat Emma was wearing. Emma deliberately twirled around and swaggered a few steps mimicking the film character. The girls were giggling at her as she paraded. She was pleased with her new feelings of confidence, realising that she didn't care about the teasing.

Mother Colette suddenly appeared in the vestry. The laughter subsided.

'Not quite school uniform,' she said to Emma, looking at her raincoat and with the girls standing watching.

'My mam got it cheap for me. She can't afford the school uniform prices. We got another baby in August,' Emma explained, quietly. Mother Colette nodded.

'I see,' she said, looking at Emma, quite caringly. She went through the chapel door. She was kind, Emma thought. Emma liked her from the start and over the last year, found her much more approachable than Mother Monica. She also discovered that Mother Colette came from a farming background in Ireland although her accent didn't reveal this as she'd lived in England for many years.

'Maybe it's why I feel okay with her,' she thought. 'The farming connection.'

Nothing more was said about the coat until she arrived home for Christmas.

'Well, was that coat all right, then?' questioned Mary, watching Emma undoing the belt fastener and taking off her coat. Emma looked at her mam.

'Mother Colette commented but didn't say I couldn't wear it. I'm quite happy with it. Don't worry, Mam. I told you that Faith was going home for Christmas to see her sister, didn't I,' she offered, changing the subject. The coat wasn't mentioned again, unlike 'Flash Harry' which continued to be her nickname for some time.

All went well in the spring term for Emma and Faith, studying hard and with little time to chat, until a problem arose for Emma. It was unintentionally instigated by their form teacher, Miss Watson. She was bubbly, outgoing and with a driving personality and was always trying to think up new ideas to stimulate the pupils. Her latest suggestion was to have formal debates to encourage pupils to discuss topics. The first time this was to take place, she chose a topic and appointed a proposer plus seconder with likewise two opposing speakers.

'Emma, you will be the proposer and Brenda, your seconder. Happy with that?' Emma's heart sank.

'I'd rather not. I'm not very good at speaking out.'

'You will be fine,' Miss Watson reassured her, whilst gazing around the form room, before naming two more speakers. 'There are four sheets of paper on my desk,' she continued. 'Pick up a copy and consult in your pairs which points you will be making so as not to have too much repetition. The rest of you will be able to ask questions on the day, after the opening speeches arguing for or against.' The bell rang and the pupils sauntered out for break time. Emma hung back.

'I can't do this,' she said to the teacher. 'I don't want to do it.'

'Nonsense. You are a clever girl. You'll be fine. It will be a good experience for you and help you grow in confidence.' Emma didn't think so.

The day arrived. At the last minute, the pupils were told that their form room was no longer the venue but that the debate was to take place in a larger room as two more classes of pupils were joining them. Emma was even more nervous.

The four speakers were at the front facing all the girls accompanied by teachers. As proposer, Emma was first to speak. She picked up her sheet and read from it. She'd prepared well but, having sat down again, never spoke another word and it fell to Brenda, her seconder, to answer all questions fired at them both. Brenda was articulate, confident and outspoken, but they lost the vote after a showing of hands. Emma, highly embarrassed, sidled out of the room as quickly as she could.

'She won't ask me again, that's for sure,' she thought, consoling herself. 'I don't think you can force people to overcome shyness, like that. Maybe she'll learn from this. I don't care.' It was days before Miss Watson caught Emma on her own.

'You tried. Maybe it was a mistake asking you,' she said. The incident wasn't referred to again, except by Laura who was sympathetic.

'I couldn't have done that,' she confided in Emma. 'I'd have probably broken down and cried.'

It was countdown to Easter. The lower fifth year pupils were ready for a break with the studying being so intense.

'You can come,' said Emma to Faith as they were collecting their books from the boarders' room. Mam says it will be fine.' She was still holding the letter that had come a day earlier than usual and she'd just skimmed through it.

'That's lovely,' Faith replied, smiling at Emma. 'I've missed not coming but I know I can't come every holiday and Rose and my uncles like to see me in some holidays. I want to tell you something, but when we're on our own. Maybe at recreation tonight.'

'It all sounds a bit mysterious,' thought Emma, as they made their way down the stairs to the main hall. 'Is everything all right?' she whispered, knowing they weren't allowed to talk.

'Yes. I just want to tell you something, but not anyone else.'

It was after evening prayers, much later in the day, when the two girls found themselves a quiet corner in the recreation hall. Faith came straight to the point.

'My mam left me a letter that she'd written when she was dying.' After this statement, Faith paused and swallowed. Emma took her hand and held it tightly whilst Faith regained her composure. 'I didn't read it at first. I couldn't. But now I like to, at times. She'd be so pleased I have a friend like you.' Emma smiled. She didn't feel she'd done much, but Faith was rather special and fit in so well into their family. 'Some of it is about my dad and that's what I want to tell you. My mam explained that my dad was a really nice guy and that as I grow older, I'll understand that sometimes things happen that are unplanned especially when two people need comfort and understanding. She says she met him when she went in August of nineteen thirty-nine, on holiday for two weeks, to Seaham on the east coast, with her girlfriend, leaving Rose with my uncles. She loved them and was fine. This was a year or so after Rose's dad died in the accident and mam had had a very tough time after the crash and following his death. I'll tell you more when we have time,' she whispered, seeing Audrey approaching them. 'It's good to be able to tell you.' There wasn't another opportunity until the following evening when Faith was able to continue her story.

The girls were sitting together at one end of the hall. The gramophone was playing. Some girls were dancing. Faith opened the letter.
'This is the bit about my dad,' she said, unfolding the letter taken from inside the book she was carrying. 'My mam says that he'd lost his mother recently and that he was an only child and he knew nothing about his dad. It had just been him and his mam. Here, you read this paragraph,' she continued, folding the page before handing it to Emma. Emma read the words, small but clearly written. Faith's mam was a tidy writer.

He introduced himself as John. At first, we met up in the evenings after he came home from his work on a farm, but he managed to take a holiday the second week. We spent the whole week together as my friend met up with a bloke and they hung out most of the time with a group of his friends. John and I spent our days going for walks together or staying at his small terraced house. John talked about his mam and their years together. He was such a kind man, Faith, as well as being tall and good looking. The last night we got carried away as we knew we wouldn't see each other

*anymore. It was weeks later when back home that I realised
I was pregnant.*

Emma stopped reading and handed the letter back to Faith.
'So that's who your dad was. Did your mam get in touch with
him again?'
'Well, yes and no,' replied Faith, placing the letter back
inside her book. 'She explains further that she decided not
to, at first, waiting till she'd come to terms with the situation.
Then, when she finally decided that she would, she wrote to
him, but the letter was returned *Not at this address.* She had
no means of knowing where he'd gone. So that was it really.
She just carried on at home and my uncles helped her. I've
never known any different sort of life.'
'So, you'll never know?'
'I suppose not. The only other bit of knowledge is that he told
my mam he was called John Cummins as that was the name
on his birth certificate, Cummins being his mother's maiden
name. His dad's name wasn't registered. All a bit of a
mystery, really.'
'How strange. I wonder where he went or if he ever found
out who his dad was.' Faith shrugged her shoulders.
'Who knows,' she stated. 'It's just weird finding this out, now.
I don't suppose I'll ever meet my dad, but it's good to hear
from my mam that he was a decent bloke. That helps me
and I'm proud of my mam. It must have been hard for her.
She had a tough life.' Faith's face crumpled.

'Come on, let's dance,' suggested Emma, pulling Faith onto
the floor. 'When we go next time to Windrush, we'll be really
good at this' she added, as they glided around the floor
weaving in and out of other girls. Emma knew the quick-step
very well as she'd spent many evenings over the winter
months with Faith and sometimes with a different partner,
dancing the quick-step, when the boarders went for
recreation after supper. She recalled her earlier efforts.
'You'll have to pull your shoulders back, Emma,' Faith
declared, one evening. The old gramophone was grinding
out music and Emma decided to give it a go. 'I'll play man
first, until you get the hang of it. My uncles have been
teaching me in our kitchen at home. They're a good laugh.
One step back and another,' she said, manoeuvring her

friend around the floor. 'See how Margaret and Maria are doing it.' Emma was stilted and slow at first, but practising night after night, she finally relaxed and was finding herself even looking forward to the evenings. 'We'll practise the waltz, too,' stated Faith. 'Once you get the hang of the different rhythms, you'll pick up other dances in no time.' 'She was right,' Emma decided, bringing herself back to the present, as the pair of them waltzed around the floor, passing comments with other dancers who came up close. It wasn't long before the bell rang, calling a halt to their fun.

The Easter holidays passed all too quickly and soon they were back at school. Faith thoroughly enjoyed her stay at Bankside, going to church on the tractor, playing cards in the evenings or having a singsong with Mary playing her banjo, a very old one given to Mary by her father. The girls went dancing once but Faith had no desire to smoke.
'I tried it with my uncles,' she informed Emma and Martha, 'and didn't enjoy it at all.' Martha spent a lot of time with a group of friends that were regulars at the village dances whilst Emma and Faith either danced occasionally when asked by a lad or they danced together. Faith enjoyed other evenings playing cards especially when Tim, who was now working full-time on a farm a few miles away but still living at home, joined them. He was a tall, dark-haired, good-looking teenager who'd just celebrated his seventeenth birthday. He joked and teased Faith over her card playing when she made mistakes, but Faith took it all in her stride, enjoying the family banter.

As in the previous year's summer term, a handful of boarders participated in the early evening trips to the swimming pool, this another joy to Emma. Even these excursions weren't without problems, as Emma recalled when writing to Martha one Saturday morning, trying to give her snippets of interesting news as so much was just routine.

It was like this. Once, we were so hungry after our session at the baths even though we'd had our bread and jam beforehand, that we decided to sneak back into the refectory on our return and raid the bread bin. It was Audrey's

suggestion. When I said, I'd rather not because we might get into trouble, she called me a little goody, goody. It's not the first time either. I don't like it when I get called that. So, I went along with the idea, but I was a bit nervous about it. The bread bin is kept to one side on a table in the refectory. The first time, the plan worked as there was no-one around and we helped ourselves. We were secretly delighted with our scheming and vowed to do this again. We didn't risk it every time, but one evening, feeling so ravenous as we ambled along the pavements to Queen Street, we decided to chance it again. After taking off our blazers and outdoor shoes in the vestry, we headed for the refectory, glancing up and down to make sure no-one was around. We slipped quietly in, closing the door behind us. Giggling a little at our audacity before busily tucking into the bread and jam and chattering unconcernedly, we failed to see the door open. We were appalled when Mother Teresa came into view. You should have seen her face! She gazed around at the six of us whilst weighing up the circumstances of this little rendezvous. None of us dared to say anything.
'What is the meaning of this?' she asked us, very sternly, you know, like they do, although normally she's quite friendly with us. You could tell that she was furious. We looked at each other and then Faith spoke, hesitantly but bravely, I thought.
'We have been to the swimming baths and we were hungry. We didn't think it would matter.' Then Mother Teresa retorted angrily.
'You will all be reported to Mother Colette,' she said, before storming out. Busily telling her tale, Emma suddenly realised that it was tea-time. *Sorry, Martha, I will have to stop but I'll tell you next time what happened after that. It wasn't so bad, actually; the punishment, I mean. Give the kids a cuddle from me. With love, Emma.*

As she was putting away her writing paper, she vividly recalled what took place later that evening. The girls were dumfounded at being found out.
'What shall we do?' Faith asked. No-one replied. In silence they quickly finished eating their bread and left the refectory. They quietly made their way up to the attic to hang their bathing costumes and wet towels along the wire lines, to dry

out ready for the next swimming lesson.
'Thank you, Audrey, for lending me your bathing costume,'
ventured Emma, as the girls were hanging up their bathers.
Audrey possessed more than one and kindly offered to lend
Emma a costume after Emma's accidently ripped when she
was taking it off after the previous trip.
'You can borrow it until you get yours mended, if you like,'
Audrey said, graciously. 'It's not my favourite but it looks
okay on you.' Emma was anxious that it was a bit see-
through but no-one else commented. She guessed she
worried unnecessarily. She was very self-conscious about
her developing figure.

After changing out of their uniform, the girls returned to the
boarders' room and informed the nun-in-charge that they'd
been swimming. Quietly, they collected their homework
books from their lockers, having placed them there after
school finished, before going swimming. Most of the
boarders were engrossed with their work and took little
notice of them. Faith and Emma sidled into seats near the
centre of the room leaving Audrey and the other three to find
empty places elsewhere. Occasionally, as the evening wore
on, they glanced furtively at each other across the tables,
waiting for the eventual summons. It came, all too soon for
Emma. She hadn't been in trouble before and feared the
consequences. At seven o'clock, the nun called out.
'Will those girls who were caught eating bread in the
refectory at a forbidden time, earlier this evening, please
report to Mother Colette's office, immediately.' The six girls
in question stood up quietly and made their way to the door,
much to the surprise of the remaining boarders who stopped
working to watch the culprits leave, hardly believing that
they'd been caught out. These six weren't known to be ones
to get into trouble.

Led by Audrey who was seated at a table nearest the door
and the first to leave the room, the girls walked to the office
of Mother Colette, only a few yards away. Audrey knocked
on the door and they waited. Emma felt sick. She wondered
if Mother Colette would tell her parents. Would she be in
trouble at home for this, as well as at school?
'Come in,' a crisp voice called out. The girls stood close

together in her small office, not knowing where to look. Mother Colette raised her eyebrows. 'I'm waiting,' she said. 'What have you to say for yourselves? I'm very surprised to see you here, Emma Holmes and you, Faith and Audrey. In fact, all of you.' She glanced at the other three and waited.

The girls tried to offer explanations, interrupting each other in their nervousness. Mother Colette held up her hand. 'Enough. I'm very disappointed in you all.' She turned her pen around and around as she considered an appropriate punishment. She acknowledged to herself that the girls had probably been very hungry to do such a thing and that that situation needed rectifying. Emma, watching the nun intently, found Mother Colette to always be fair and was a little sad that she'd let her down. 'You will take your meals, breakfast, tea and supper, to the far end of the refectory where the day pupils have dinner, for three days; each of you at a separate table and you will eat in silence, reflecting on your misdemeanour. Now return to your studies.' They sheepishly walked out, not knowing if they were supposed to say anything.
'Well, that's not so bad,' whispered Audrey, as they were quietly walking back the few yards to the boarders' room. 'At least we can smile at each other across the tables from our isolated seating arrangement. It means we go last to get our breakfast and cups of tea, but never mind. Cheer up, Emma, it could have been worse.' Emma nodded, relieved that it was over. She'd seen one or two other boarders at the far end of the refectory in punishment, on occasions.
'It's a pity I won't be able to take a book to read, but that isn't allowed,' she thought, resignedly.

A bright spot for Emma at the end of this term was at the final assembly in the school hall before breaking up. It was a special occasion when book prizes were distributed and much to her surprise, her name was called out. She walked onto the stage and was handed her prize by Mother Margaret who congratulated her on her consistently good work, the reason she had received the prize. Mother Superior always attended these special occasions. It was only when back in her form room that Emma had a quick look at her prize entitled *Julius Caesar and the Life of*

William Shakespeare. She wasn't sure when she would read it but knew her parents would be pleased.

The summer holidays finally arrived.
'See you in six weeks,' Emma called out before stepping from the bus and waving to the boarders staying on.
'Another year finished,' she thought. She was looking forward to Faith joining her in a couple of weeks. Meanwhile, she knew Martha would have plenty of 'boys' news for her. 'But where is she,' she thought, after crossing the road and stepping onto the cart track leading across the moor. She gazed into the distance but saw no-one. 'She said she'd meet me so that we could have a good chat. She must have been delayed.' She walked some yards across the track before seeing Martha emerging from behind a clump of heather. 'Why did you hide?' she questioned, feeling very puzzled.
'I didn't want your friends on the bus to see me in my working overalls,' replied Martha, looking at Emma's smart uniform.
'Well, it wouldn't have bothered me,' replied Emma, defensively. 'Did she think I was ashamed of her?' she wondered. 'Honestly, Martha. You need never think I'm ashamed of you. I couldn't care less. You're my sister. I've been so looking forward to hearing all the news. I hope you have something exciting to tell me.'

Emma dwelt on this late at night, before falling asleep. Martha, with her bubbly, out-going personality, her deep brown eyes and curly black hair, was very attractive. She was an excellent dancer and very popular with the local lads. Tom described Martha has having plenty of 'oomph' and referred to his two older daughters as the substance and the shadow, as Martha was a little on the plump side and Emma, with her long legs, now taller than Martha, was almost skinny.
'He's right,' thought Emma. 'I am her shadow. I hang around with her at dances and sometimes she finds me a ride home with someone if she's fixed up with a lad.' On occasions, to go to dances, the girls used the taxi, run by one of the locals, sharing it with others from the village after walking the mile to the moor track end to catch it. To get home, they often

made other arrangements, such as a ride on the back of motor bikes or squashed together with other dancers in the back of a car belonging to one of the lads. Martha never had any difficulty getting a ride for the pair of them. Emma admired her sister.

It was hay time again. A treat for Emma, wearing a pair of Martha's overalls, was when she joined her sister to help in the fields, forking the hay into haycocks, alongside Tim, as he'd taken a couple of days holiday to help his dad. The sun was blazing down and the work was continuous until Tom spied Mary, coming down the field, pushing the old, rickety, black pram with its patched corners on the hood. Miriam, propped up on a cushion, was gazing around whilst Jacob, on spying his dad, set off running across the stubble. 'Time for a cup of tea, lasses,' Tom called as he and Tim stuck their hay forks in the haycock and began walking across to where the girls were working. They all sat down

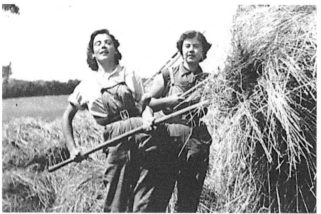

Hay time at Bankside - Emma (left) and Martha

under the hedgerow, away from the spiky stubble but feeling the warmth of the sun blazing down. Tom pulled out his woodbines and matches from the pocket of his jacket that he'd left by the hedgerow and lit up a cigarette, before handing them to his girls. They each took out a woodbine and lit up, the grey smoke swirling and rising amongst the sun rays. Tim wasn't interested in having a smoke.

'Mark and Amy didn't want to come,' stated Mary, parking the pram safely so that the glare of the sun wasn't in Miriam's face. She took out cups from the basket and each person held one whilst she poured the tea. There were biscuits for those who wanted one. Emma loved sitting with her dad and mam, smoking and chatting, enjoying the cigarette and thought that it seemed such a grown-up thing to do.

'Not a cloud in sight,' she thought, gazing up at clear blue sky, puffing on her woodbine and thinking how far removed this was from the discipline of boarding school. 'It's so tranquil and still.' She quietly watched the little black beetles scurrying around in the grass until Miriam, started getting restless, disturbed her thoughts with her shouts for attention. Stubbing out her cigarette on the parched ground, Emma stood up and began rocking the pram a little to settle Miriam. 'You are beautiful with those big brown eyes and cute little nose. Even your lips are a perfect rosebud colour,' she thought, smiling at her baby sister.

'I'll take her back,' Mary said to Emma, as she got to her feet and picked up the basket. 'Collect the cups for me, please, will you. I miss your help, but getting the hay cocked is so important. Then it will be getting it in before the weather breaks.' Emma smiled. She normally helped Mary but was delighted to be outside.

'Well, who's this then,' exclaimed Tom, staring into the distance at a figure emerging. 'It's Jack.'
'I thought another pair of hand might help,' Jack said, approaching the family. 'Morning Mary. And how are you, little smiler?' he said to Miriam, leaning into the pram. 'She is a little smasher, isn't she. Now, lasses, going dancing again, are you on Tuesday? It's at Windrush, isn't it.' The girls nodded. 'I've been telling Greg about the dances. He might go.'
'Is he the lad that's hanging around your place sometimes when dad and I come?' questioned Martha. 'That tall lad with black hair?'
'Aye, that's Greg. He lives up the dales and earns himself a bit of money helping me. He's a good worker, clever as well, apparently. He's going to Askham Bryan College in another year, he hopes.'

'Emma,' interrupted Tom, 'give Uncle Jack your hayfork and you go off with your mam and give her a hand.' Emma handed over the fork and whispered in Martha's ear. 'Sounds promising. Let's hope he goes.' Martha knew she was referring to Greg and the dance. She grinned in acknowledgement and returned to the hard work in the hay field.

'All done up for tonight, are you,' Tom said on Tuesday evening, admiring his daughters. Both were wearing black taffeta, swirling skirts, Emma with a red blouse and Martha, a white one. They were pretty girls, with their black curly hair and lips enhanced with bright red lipstick.
'I'd take a bit of that lipstick off, if I were you,' said Tom. 'You don't want it too bright.' He was proud of his two older girls and long since accepted the regular home-perming sessions in the farmhouse kitchen. 'Enjoy yourselves,' he called, as they left. Tim wasn't interested in going dancing and was happily teaching Mark to skilfully play draughts.

Tom turned his attention to the lads. 'Now, Mark,' he said, interrupting the game. 'Your mam and I have discussed your options for school in September. We know you don't want to go to a boarding school. Tim wasn't particularly happy at Whitby. How about the Catholic grammar school in Middlesbrough? I can contact Uncle Sam to see if one of his family has a spare room where you could stay during the week. What do you think?' He paused, waiting for Mark's response. Mark raised his head and gazed at his dad with his big brown eyes and nodded. He'd passed his eleven plus exam and talks had been going on for days about which school to go to.
'Yes, Dad. That sounds okay,' he said, unenthusiastically. 'At least I'll get home for weekends. It should be all right.' With that, Mark returned his concentration to considering his next move on the draughts board.
'Well, that's settled then,' replied Tom, looking over at Mary. 'You'll write to Sam, will you, Mary? Did the girls say how they were getting home tonight?'
'I'll write tomorrow and no, they didn't, but they'll be fine. Martha will sort something out. They were both so excited about going.'

The girls, meanwhile, were eagerly anticipating their night out as they were making their way over the moor to go to the dance.

'It's a pity Faith isn't here,' commented Emma to Martha, on arriving in the village. 'Maybe she'll make the next one.' Entering the hall, the girls joined others lining one side, as was customary, eyeing up the lads sitting on the other side of the room. A few grown-ups were standing at the back catching up, no doubt, on farming news. It was quite a community gathering when a dance was held at Windrush. 'He's there,' whispered Martha to Emma, 'almost halfway down the room. Can you see him. He's the one with the black hair and tall and slim, wearing a grey, striped shirt, the lad I saw at Uncle Jack's farm. I'm sure of it.' Emma nodded. 'So that's Greg.'

'And guess who else,' Martha continued. 'Paul is further up near the top of the hall. He's got a dark blue shirt on. The blond lad. I think it's going to be a good night.'

Eventually the band struck up and the MC (Master of Ceremonies) invited everyone to take up their partner for a quickstep. Lads slowly made their way across the floor to choose a girl to ask for a dance. Martha could see Paul inching his way across towards her. He caught her eye and smiled as he reached her. She stood up and together they joined many other young couples gliding around the dance floor. Emma waited a while, watching the dancers and wondering if anyone would ask her.

'Would you like to dance?' the voice brought Emma back to the present.

'Sorry, I was day-dreaming. Yes, I would, thank you,' she replied, standing up and looking into the eyes of this good-looking lad.

'I'm Greg,' he informed her. 'Your Uncle Jack told me to look out for you and your sister,' he continued, as they made their way to the centre of the dance floor. 'You're very much alike, aren't you?' he added, a little later. Emma nodded, concentrating on the steps and feeling quite chuffed to be gliding around the floor with this young man. She was so pleased that she'd practised at school, even though she'd taken some ragging about being round-shouldered and hunched-back.

'They even suggested I walk around the hall with a book on my head,' she reminisced.

Faith arrived a week later, delighted to be at Bankside again. She entertained the little ones and spent evenings joining in if there was a singsong. Cards were fun, especially when Tim chose to play.
'I think you fancy him,' Emma said to her jokingly, one day.
'Don't be daft,' replied Faith, but couldn't hide the fact that she was blushing. 'I enjoy his company, but that's all,' she insisted. The weeks passed quickly.
'There's another dance at Windrush next Tuesday before we go back,' Emma told Faith one morning. 'Shall we go? Have you anything suitable to wear?'
'I brought a pretty summer dress just in case,' replied Faith.
'Will your mam and dad be going?'
'Dad might if Uncle Jack goes, as I know they like to talk.'
Tom later told them that he'd been visiting Jack and that Jack would take them in his van and stay a while at the dance.
'I'll come as well, but I'll be leaving with Jack. You'll have to get yourselves home,' he added.

The evening was a great success as both Paul and Greg turned up. Faith, who was introduced to them, was spotted by the locals as an outsider and a couple of lads were pleased to invite her onto the floor for a dance. Jack and Tom gave each the girls a dance before leaving.
'Mind you're not too late,' were their dad's parting words before leaving with Jack. As they pulled away, Tom looked at his brother.
'You're very serious. Got a problem?'
'Not really. It's just that lass, Faith. Emma's friend. She seems familiar, but I hadn't met her before she started visiting Bankside. Whilst we were dancing, she was telling me how much she loved coming to stay, especially since her mam died over three years ago. No mention of a dad. Apparently, she lives with three bachelor uncles and an older sister, Rose. No wonder she enjoys being with your family, Tom. There's something about her that's niggling away at the back of my mind. Maybe it will come to me.'

Autumn to Summer 1956

After a long hot summer of work and leisure, Faith and
Emma, on returning to boarding school, were soon
immersed into a heavy workload of studying, but there were
lighter moments. Becoming more confident and a little
rebellious, some of the older girls broke the rules in the
dormitory by visiting friends for a chat or to share food,
always late and well after night prayers. Even Emma who'd
never dared to do this in the earlier years, was now taking
risks occasionally and sneaking into Faith's cubicle, further
down the garden side. Unfortunately, Rita was caught
visiting another girl in her cubicle, without permission,
breaking two rules, the other of no talking in the dormitory.
As a punishment, her bed was dragged out into the central
aisle for all to see as they walked in and out of the dormitory.
It had to remain there for three days and nights.

Earlier, on the second of these three days, Rita had been
teasing Emma and although Emma joined in the banter, she
decided to get her own back by playing a trick on Rita.
'But what can I do,' she thought, sitting on her bed, that
evening. Then spying her facecloth hanging on the bar
under her sink, she soaked it in water, squeezed out the
excess, and stealthily walked around to the dormitory
entrance. Mother Teresa was not at her table. Rita was not
in her bed. 'Probably getting washed,' thought Emma. She
walked quickly to Rita's bed and placed the damp cloth
under her top sheet. 'Just in time,' she thought, as Mother
Teresa returned to her station. The short, nightly prayers
followed, led by the nun and responded to by the boarders.
Lights went out and all was quiet until, suddenly, there was a
scream as Rita, having crawled into bed, discovered the wet
cloth.

Lights went on and Mother Teresa, after investigating, called
out.
'Will the person responsible for placing a wet facecloth in
Rita's bed, please come here immediately.' Emma
reluctantly got out of bed, put on her dressing gown and
made her way to the centre aisle, to own up. 'You!'
exclaimed Mother Teresa, unbelievingly. 'You, I will report to

Mother Colette tomorrow. Now go and get some dry sheets from the linen cupboard and help Rita make her bed.' Emma did as instructed. Together, they made the bed, whilst smiling at each other. Neither were unduly upset.

When Emma returned to the dormitory the following evening, her bed was missing from her cubicle. She wandered around to speak with Mother Teresa.
'You will be sleeping in the junior dormitory for three nights. I don't know what you were thinking of, doing such a thing.'
'Makes sense,' surmised Emma, going back to her cubicle. 'It wouldn't be much of a punishment putting me next to Rita and it would block the aisle, too.' When ready for bed and just before lights went out, Emma made her way to the junior dormitory. It was embarrassing, but the young girls did not speak to her as they were keeping the rules. It was further embarrassing the following evening when Mother Margaret paid a visit to check on one of the young boarders who was unwell. She glanced at Emma but said nothing.
'You were stupid to do that,' Faith remarked, the day following the incident.
'I know, but I'm not that bothered,' replied Emma. 'It was a laugh. Rita saw the funny side afterwards.'

A few weeks later, Emma was caught talking at a forbidden time and without permission. She was told to spend two days in isolation at the other end of the refectory at mealtimes, excluding weekday dinners when it was not possible as the refectory filled up with day girls. It came as a surprise to some of the boarders as Emma wasn't noted for breaking rules.
'Must be my rebellious streak surfacing,' Emma whispered to Faith as she passed her in the breakfast queue for the tea urn. She pondered on this as she returned to her solitary place. 'Maybe it is because I am confident these days and academically doing well that I don't care as much. It's quite good, feeling different. So unlike my earlier years,' she mused.

Mealtimes also had some lighter moments. To pass the time, after finishing eating and waiting for everyone else to end their meal, as grace after meals was said only when

everyone was ready, the girls amused themselves by playing 'spin the knife.' It seemed a daft game to Emma when younger, but now that her interest in boys was developing, she was enjoying it more. Spinning the knife meant trying to discover what kind of person one would become, or who one would marry and even how many children one would have. As the knife was spinning, one of the girls quietly said the words of an occupation of a future husband: *tinker, tailor, soldier, sailor, rich man, poor man, beggar man, thief, doctor, lawyer, merchant, chief.* Whatever word was being uttered when the knife stopped, that was a prediction of the fate of the girl to whom the knife was pointing. Descriptions on the appearance of this fellow, were chanted: *tall, dark and handsome; fair, fat and forty.* The bride's dress was described: *silk, satin, velvet, rags.* Predictions on numbers of children were added. The girls giggled. It was a stupid game but caused much laughter.
'I think, Emma, that you will marry either a doctor or a farmer,' piped up one of the girls. Emma grinned.
'I'm not sure about a doctor,' she commented. 'Maybe a farmer.'

At half-term, Faith decided to go home for some quiet study time as she knew there would not be an opportunity at Bankside with all the goings on. Emma enjoyed the break away from her books. The studying and revision were relentless, building up to mock exams in the spring term, before the real ones in the summer term. The senior girls knuckled down and worked hard until the Christmas break which passed very quickly. Martha and Emma managed a couple of Saturday night dances in the next village but without Faith, who, as usual, went home to spend it with her sister and uncles.

Martha was meeting up with Paul more often, but Emma hadn't seen Greg since the summer holidays. He wasn't at the first dance this holiday, but there were plenty of other lads asking Emma onto the dance floor. One of them was Andy. She thought that he was quite canny and although shy and quiet, was a lovely dancer. His brown hair was cut very short as he was in the army. She knew he was keen on her because, having asked her once, he was quick off the mark getting across the floor to ask her again. He talked a lot about his home life but little about the army. Emma reciprocated with tales about the farm and that she went to a boarding school in Scarborough.

'We're all piling into the taxi tonight to get home,' Martha informed her over the tea break, halfway through the evening.

'That's a relief,' thought Emma, knowing that if Andy asked her how she was getting home, she had a genuine plan that didn't involve him as she wasn't overly interested in him seeing her home.

Greg turned up at the next weekend dance. He seemed pleased to see Emma again. They had studies in common especially with Greg hoping to further his education at Askham Bryan College. They were very relaxed in each other's company. She was glad that Andy didn't appear to complicate matters.

'How about we have a run out to Scarborough on our motorbikes and take Emma back to boarding school?' Greg suggested to Paul, as the four of them stood in a huddle towards the end of the evening. Emma grinned. She loved riding pillion. She didn't think her parents would mind either. It would save her bus fare.

'Will you really?' she asked, her face lightening up with excitement at such a thought.

'I don't see why we shouldn't,' commented Paul.

A few days later, the two lads turned up at Bankside to pick up the girls.

'I'll tie your case on,' Greg said to Emma. 'It's not my bike, you know. It's my brother's but he lets me borrow it. I have to look after it though.'

'Ride carefully,' called Mary, as the boys revved up their bikes and pulled away. She watched from the doorway, holding Miriam in her arms, with Jacob and Amy standing, one at each side, waving until the bikes were out of sight. 'How quickly they grow up,' she thought, feeling a little sad.

As they approached Scarborough, Emma started shouting directions to Greg, raising her voice above the noise of the motorbikes as Paul and Martha were following closely behind. They finally turned into Queen Street and Emma pointed out to Greg the enormous red brick building, where he pulled to a halt with Paul close behind. The lads got off their motor bikes and gazed. They noticed the large wooden doors with a little spy hole and a ring for a handle, but mostly, they gazed at the metal spiked bars along the length of the front of the building.

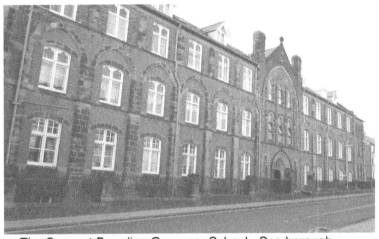

The Convent Boarding Grammar School - Scarborough

'It is huge. It looks like a prison,' voiced Greg, in amazement. 'It doesn't look like a school at all, or a convent.' Emma laughed.
'They have beautiful grounds and tennis courts around the back,' she said, turning towards Greg. 'Anyway, thanks for the ride. It was great. I'll see you next holiday.' He untied her case from the bike and when handing it to her, gave her a quick kiss. Emma blushed. She was worried someone might see them. She said goodbye to Martha and Paul, before walking up to the convent doors. 'Go,' she called to them, waving them away. The bikes roared as they disappeared down the street. 'I can't wait to tell Faith,' she thought, gleefully.

The letters started arriving and Mother Colette gave Emma an enquiring look when handing her the fourth of the week. Emma had no real interest in Andy and was thinking that maybe she shouldn't have told him which boarding school she went to. The letters were very short. She guessed he was lonely away from his family in Ireland. Emma wrote a letter that night, whilst in her cubicle, putting in a bit of chit-chat about school and suggesting that maybe he didn't write quite so often as the nun in charge was giving her some funny looks. The following day, Emma gave the letter to Laura with money for a stamp, having kept some back for just such an occasion, when handing in her purse. She re-read Andy's letters too. They were only a few sentences long.

'He doesn't have much to say, poor lad. He probably doesn't have anything to write about. He said they were going abroad soon. He'll probably stop writing then,' were her thoughts. She felt quite sorry for him but her interest in boys lay elsewhere. Receiving Andy's letter reminded her of when she'd written to Martin whilst recovering from German measles. 'But that's almost two years ago,' she thought, 'and he never wrote back again. Not that it matters,' she realised, as it was some time since Emma had given a thought to Martin.

An exciting invitation early in the spring term, was when Mrs Carruthers, the PE teacher and swimming tutor, asked if any of the upper fifth girls would like to participate in professionally taught ballroom dancing classes. The parents of one of the day girls, whom, she explained, were members of *The Empire Society of Teachers of Dancing*, were offering to take classes one evening a week in the school hall. They were both accomplished dancers and ran a dancing school in the town. Medals and certificates were to be awarded to those who reached certain standards.

'I'll be there, too,' Mrs Carruthers stated. 'It would be great to have a good number of you attending, to show appreciation of such generosity as they are not charging any fees. It is their way of supporting the school,' she explained. 'Put your names on the sheet of paper as you leave, if you are interested.' She also informed them that Mother Colette approved, provided studies were not neglected.

Emma wrote her name, hoping that Faith would also be taking up this offer.

'Free instructions from a professional,' she thought. 'This is amazing.' It was even more so, when finding out the names of the dances that she was about to be taught. She knew the Waltz but was intrigued to read Veleta, Boston Two Step, Royal Empress Tango and Latchford Schottische.
After a very rushed half-term of four days at Bankside, Emma and Faith came back to constant studying and pressure from teachers to keep revising for the mock exams. It was a heavy schedule, but the dancing lessons were providing some light relief.

'Emma, your deportment is shocking. We must work on that. If you can hold yourself more elegantly, you may reach the gold medal standard, as your dancing is good,' explained Mrs Carruthers, at the beginning of a session, one evening. 'You have grasped the Tango well and the Waltz and Veleta. We need a little more practise on the other two, but even with those, you have made good progress. It is your deportment that is a concern. You need to relax more.' She glanced at her notes sheet. 'Faith, we are pleased with your dancing and you are very graceful on the dance floor. Well done.' Mrs Carruthers went through the names of each pupil, giving advice or criticism as well as encouragement. 'You are all doing remarkably well, especially those of you who were clueless about ballroom dancing when we began these lessons. You should be pleased with yourselves, no matter what standard you achieve. Four more weeks and you will be taking the exams,' she concluded. The two instructors were listening, quite aware of the different levels the girls were reaching, having spent some time discussing their progress with the schoolteacher, after six weeks of classes. Emma was thrilled.
'It's all that practising we've been doing,' she said to Faith, pleased that it looked promising for them both to gain a gold medal.

The dancing exams were imminent. Mrs Carruthers organised an extra lesson or two, to help those who were struggling, but Emma declined.
'I think I'll just stick to the one evening's lesson,' she said to Faith. 'Mrs Carruthers said it wasn't necessary for me and there's no advantage like missing the weekly walk, now it's

not obligatory for our year.' Mother Colette was allowing the upper fifth form boarders extra revision time, in place of the customary daily walk. This was especially helpful to Emma and Faith in compensating for time taken out for the weekly dancing lesson.

On the day itself, the adjudicators and instructors were already in place in the hall when the girls trooped in with their teacher. Emma was very tense and felt a little sick. Mrs Carruthers, along with the two instructors, each led a pupil onto the dance floor. She awaited her turn and was glad that it was their teacher who was partnering her. She would have been even more nervous had it been one of the instructors. The music began. Her teacher held Emma tightly and almost pushed her around the dance floor but in a manner that enabled her to correctly perform the steps.
'Relax,' she whispered, but Emma couldn't. She was stiff and tense. However, she felt that her footwork was good and she didn't think she'd made any glaring mistakes.
'I'm glad that's over,' said Faith, as they were leaving the hall. 'We can't do anything more now except wait for the results in a few weeks. One thing less to worry about.'
Emma agreed.

As well as sitting mock exams in March, the Catholics took the Conference of Catholic Colleges Religious Examination, well ahead of the other GCEs in June.
'And what did you put for the question about what was the cornerstone of the faith?' asked Faith, as the two girls left the exam room together.
'Marriage,' answered Emma, 'as I wasn't sure.' Faith smiled.
'I don't think that's right. I put The Resurrection.'
'Oh dear. You're probably right,' replied Emma, woefully.
'Don't tell Mother Colette, will you. She won't be happy.'
Whispering, as they walked along the corridor, they almost bumped into the headmistress.
'How was it, girls? Did you manage all the questions? You look a bit glum, Emma.' It was Faith who responded.
'It was all right, I think. I seemed to make a good shot at each question.'
'Well, we'll find out when the results come in, won't we. No slowing down though. Keep up the revision,' Mother Colette

replied, before continuing to walk on, in the opposite direction. Emma sighed.
'I'm getting sick of studying. I can't wait to leave school.'

A couple of weeks before the end of the spring term, Emma was in a dilemma. She was re-reading part of a long, newsy letter from Martha. They were both invited to an eighteenth birthday party of a friend of Martha's. *Please try and come*, wrote Martha. *It will be such fun. See if you can get permission. Uncle Jack visited yesterday and told me that he thinks Greg has been invited too. That will please you.* Emma desperately wanted to go especially as it was her first adult party.

Taking courage in both hands, she approached Mother Colette after night prayers in chapel.
'Yes, Emma,' Mother Colette said, as Emma hovered around waiting for the others to go to recreation. Emma was as tall as the nun and as they faced each other, she explained her request.
'It's a very special occasion. I've been invited along with my sister.' Emma knew other older boarders obtained permission for trips home at the weekends but there had to be a good reason. Mother Colette pondered. She was diffident in her reply, obviously not keen. It was hardly a serious reason to disappear for two days especially in the middle of mock exams. On the other hand, she knew Emma was working extremely hard and had already sat most of hers. The matter was left in the open. On Sunday, when purses were available for buying sweets, Emma remembered to keep out enough money for her bus fare. The party was the following Saturday and she was determined to go.

On the Friday, the day before the party, Emma told Faith of her plan in case anyone asked where she was over the weekend. She didn't want to cause concern because of her absence.
'Don't tell anyone why I've gone home, though,' she insisted. 'If they ask, tell them I've spoken with Mother Colette.'
'Have a lovely time, then,' voiced Faith, before they went their separate ways to lessons. Immediately after the bell

rang, signalling the end of the last lesson of the day, Emma quickly took her books to the boarders' room and returning to the vestry, put on her coat and shoes and sneaked out through the front doors as quietly as she could. No-one was around. She walked through the streets of Scarborough to the bus station and waited some time before her bus arrived. She climbed on and walked up the aisle to near the back. She had no luggage but knew Martha would lend her some suitable clothes.

'I've done it,' she thought, gleefully. 'Wait till Martha sees me.'

Two hours later and she was back home at Bankside. Martha was delighted.

'How did you get permission? Did you ask Mother Colette?'

'I did and she didn't exactly say yes but she didn't say no either. So, I came.' They giggled.

'It's going to be great,' stated Martha. 'I'm so glad you're here.'

It wasn't until Emma was standing at the bus stop on the Sunday afternoon, that she began to worry. She knew she had to report back to Mother Colette as soon as she returned. That was the rule. At this moment, a car pulled up. The driver wound down his window and asked where she was going.

'Scarborough.'

'That's where I'm going. I can take you if you like.' Emma hesitated but he seemed okay and she was in her school uniform. He'd know she was a schoolgirl.

'I'll save my bus fare, too,' she thought. 'Thank you,' she replied, opening the car door and climbing onto the front passenger seat. 'This is fun,' she thought. 'A ride back to school in a car.' She recalled the last time she'd been taken in a car to the convent which was when their parish priest at Windrush took her with her parents for her interview. 'And haven't I changed, since then. I'm so much more confident,' she thought, feeling pleased with herself.

'So which school do you attend?' the driver asked. Emma looked at him. He had dark hair, sleeked back and was quite pleasant to look at, she thought. Probably about the same

age as her dad. A bit stockier though. Tom was tall with no excess weight on him and Emma was built like him.
'The convent grammar school in Queen Street. I'm a boarder there.' The conversation flowed. They had an excellent discussion about Maths especially Algebra, a subject Emma enjoyed. It seemed no time at all before they were approaching Scarborough.
'How about a nice cup of tea before I take you to your school?' her driver said, as he drove along the sea front. 'There is plenty of time.'
'Yes, thank you. That would be nice,' replied Emma, not knowing how to refuse after he'd kindly given her a lift, but she was beginning to feel a little apprehensive. They parked outside what Emma thought was a rather grand hotel. Her companion led her inside where they sat down at one of the small tables in a large type of open room. A waitress took their order, tea for two and buttered scones.
'All very posh,' thought Emma, as she gazed around at the splendid décor.

Conversation was a little stilted, as Emma felt uneasy. She just wanted to get back to the convent. Finally, they were on their way and Emma began feeling less anxious. The man pulled his car up in Thomas Street, a small back street leading to Queen Street. Emma turned to thank him when the car stopped.
'How about a nice grown-up kiss then, before you go,' he said, smiling at her. For a second, Emma froze, before grabbing the door handle, getting out and running full pelt down Thomas Street, around the corner into Queen Street and up to the convent doors. She looked back down the street, but no-one was there. She was gasping for breath as she heard the bell ringing.
'Thank God for that,' she thought, dreading that he might have followed her. The convent door opened. She stepped inside, still feeling shocked and shaky at the man's request.

After taking off her coat and changing her shoes, she made her way upstairs to Mother Colette's office to report back. Nervousness, at the thought of facing the nun, was increasing as she climbed each step to the second floor. Emma knocked tentatively on Mother Colette's door.

'Come in.' She stepped inside. The head mistress, whose
desk was covered in exercise books that she was marking,
put down her pen and turned to face Emma.
'I'm back,' Emma volunteered, sheepishly, still shaken by the
earlier incident. 'Thank you for letting me go.'
'Did you enjoy your weekend at home?'
'Yes, I did, very much, thank you. I went to the party with my
sister Martha.'
'I don't remember saying that you could go home, you know.'
'Well, when I asked, you didn't say no. So, I thought it would
be all right,' Emma replied, quietly. She hoped that didn't
sound too cheeky.
'I had intended to discuss the matter further with you, but
now that it has taken place, we will leave it this time,' the nun
replied, a serious tone to her voice. 'Make sure you work
extra hard to compensate for the time lost.' Emma nodded.
'Thank you,' she replied, gratefully, as she left the room.
Feeling so relieved, she wanted to skip out but that would
have been unladylike. She thought that Mother Colette was
a very understanding and kind person. She liked her.

With mock exams finally over, the boarders, especially the
upper fifth formers, were eagerly awaiting the Easter
holidays.
'It's the last holiday before the big exams,' stated Emma to
Faith. 'Are you coming for both weeks at Easter?'
'I'm undecided,' she replied. 'Maybe I will come for a few
days and then go home to study. I'll get more revision done
at my place.'
'I think you're right. Why not come the second week of the
holiday and we'll enjoy some time relaxing before going
back?' Faith thought that a good plan and arrived at
Bankside on a Saturday, giving her more than a week on the
farm before the girls returned to boarding school.
'Two Sundays with rides on the tractor to church,' she
thought, feeling immensely pleased about that.

Outside church the next day, after Mass, Jack Netherfield
chatted to Mary, with Miriam in her arms and Jacob by her
side, whilst the girls hovered around. He asked the girls
about school before leaving the little group to join Tom to
walk up the village for a pint at the local pub. Martha was

away staying overnight with her friend after a dance. The other Holmes children had been to the earlier Mass, walking both ways to church. Tom only stayed a short while in the pub, before joining Mary who was waiting outside after having been to the village shop for The Farmers Weekly and some sweets for the children. It was later that Tom managed to have a quiet word with Mary.

'Jack wondered if you could find out about Faith. He didn't want to say much in the pub, but he may call in some time for a chat.'

'What do you mean, find out about Faith?'

'Just about her parents. Their names, he said. He was a bit vague, but he's got something on his mind. It's been bothering him since he was introduced to Faith. I don't know what his problem is.'

'How strange. I suppose I can ask Emma. Maybe she knows. Faith's mother died, you know. I've never heard her mention a dad. I'll see what I can do.'

It was later, on the Sunday afternoon, before Mary was able to speak to Emma alone, Faith having offered to take Miriam out in the pram for a walk, with Jacob and Amy tagging along. Mary didn't mention Jack but tried to sound casual, as if she was just being curious, when asking Emma.

'I'll ask Faith if it's all right to tell you,' said Emma, 'but I'm sure she won't mind you knowing. She might like to tell you, herself. She looks on this as her second home and says you are always so kind to her.' Later in the evening, when they were in the sitting room getting ready for bed, Emma mentioned to Faith, the conversation with Mary.

'I don't mind your mam and dad knowing. I'll tell them tomorrow night when the little ones are not there.' The following evening, Tom and Mary listened sympathetically whilst Faith told her story.

The next day, Jack visited the Holmes family. The children were outside playing with Emma and Faith keeping a motherly eye on them. Mary made Jack a cup of tea and took the opportunity to tell him about Faith's parents.

'What's the matter, Jack? You seem a bit disturbed by what I've told you. What is your interest?' Jack looked at her.

'I'm trying to sort something out in my mind. She reminds me of someone that I was introduced to some years ago and I want to clarify something. I think I might know who her dad is, but I wouldn't want to give Faith any wrong information. I need to be absolutely certain. Are you sure she said that the holiday took place in August, nineteen thirty-nine?' Mary nodded, very surprised at Jack's explanation. 'Thanks for this, Mary. It really helps.'

The conversation changed as Tom walked in and the two blokes went off to look at one of Tom's cows that was ailing. It was later in the evening when Tom passed on a message to Emma.
'Jack wants to come around and have a chat with you and Faith before you go back to school. He says he'll call in Wednesday evening.' Emma looked at her dad.
'Did he tell you why?' Tom hesitated, not sure how much to say.
'Not exactly, but I think he has some information for Faith. It's nothing to worry about.'
'I'll make sure we're in,' Emma replied but she couldn't possibly imagine what Jack wanted to tell Faith and she was very curious.

It was quite late on Wednesday evening when Jack made his appearance, wearing a tweed jacket and looking very spruced up. He wore a small-checked blue and white shirt and a pair of brown corduroys. He was clean-shaven with his dark brown hair neatly combed. He smiled and said hello to the girls, his blue eyes twinkling under his bushy eyebrows. Tom came in, having finished for the evening.
'You're looking a bit smart tonight, Jack. What's the occasion?'
'I just thought I'd make an effort for these two charming young ladies,' Jack replied, with a grin.
'Do you fancy a pint, then? I've got a barrel of beer in this year, for when we're hay-timing. We could open it now.'
'Thanks, Tom. I will have one.' Tom disappeared into the dairy to get the drinks. Mary was hustling the younger children off to bed, Miriam having been settled earlier. Tim disappeared to go rabbit hunting, one of his favourite pass-times.
'Martha's probably staying in Whitby until the last bus as she

was meeting up with her friend. If you want a chat, Jack, now's the time,' Mary said to him, quietly, having come back downstairs. 'It isn't often it's so peaceful in here. It probably won't last either,' she added, smiling at him.'

Tom handed his brother a pint, before sitting down in his armchair opposite Mary on her rocking chair. He lit up a cigarette. Jack pulled out one of the wooden chairs from the kitchen table, joining the girls.
'Well, Jack? You have something to show Faith, you said,' Tom stated, opening up the conversation. Jack gazed around, resting his eyes on Faith.
'Yes, it's you I really want to talk to, Faith. I don't mean to upset you and I hope I'm doing the right thing by telling you.' He paused. The rest of them stayed silent; Emma wondered what was coming. Faith looked particularly troubled, puzzled as to what on earth he could possibly want to tell her. Jack took a drink from his glass, before starting again. 'Don't worry. It's nothing bad. To begin with, when I first met you, Faith, I was flummoxed. You seemed familiar as if I'd seen you before, but I'd never seen you until Emma brought you to Bankside. I put it to the back of my mind but each time I met you after that, something was niggling me about you and I decided to make a few enquiries to get to the facts. You'll understand better, what I'm on about, as I explain. I asked Tom if he knew anything about your parents. Remember, Tom, when we were in the pub after church. You said you'd ask Mary.' Tom nodded

'I remember being surprised when Tom asked me if I knew who Faith's parents were and that it was you who wanted to know.' Mary voiced. 'It seemed so strange, but I questioned Emma without referring to you and she said she'd mention it to Faith. You were happy to tell us, weren't you Faith. Where's this going, Jack?' Faith looked surprised.
'I didn't know it was you who'd asked,' she said, 'not that I mind as I expected Tom to tell you, with you two being so close, but why did you want to know?' Jack took a drink from his pint glass.

They all remained silent, waiting for him to speak.
'I'm sorry Faith. I didn't feel I could approach you directly, but

I had good reason to ask, as you will find out. After I was given the information, it seemed to me that I'm right in what I think.' Jack took his cigarettes out from the pocket of his jacket and lit up, taking a long drag. 'Before I came back here to find my dad, I lived in Seaham with my mam and my stepdad although I wasn't particularly close to him. I was only in my twenties when my mam died and this left me very downcast, feeling I had no-one. I did meet up regularly with a group of lads though, mostly in a pub. One evening, John, who usually joined us, introduced us to this lass. She was called Rose and she'd come with her friend to Seaham for a couple of weeks holiday. It was August. She'd lost her husband a year or so earlier in an accident. Her friend teamed up with another lad in our group and spent time with us, but we hardly saw John after that as he spent all his time with Rose. He told us after the lasses had gone back home that Rose was the gentlest, most caring person that he'd ever known.'

Faith was listening intently. Jack paused, before continuing, choosing his words very carefully and softening his voice, not knowing quite how Faith was taking this. 'John and Rose met up in the pub once more and someone took a photo of her and her friend with some of us lads including John. A few weeks later, I was given a copy, seeing as I'm on it, and I've kept it all these years.' He paused and pulled an old envelope out of his pocket and from it took a small, rather faded, black and white photograph. He slid it across the table to Faith. 'See, that's Rose and that's John,' he said, pointing them out. 'That's John Cummins.'

For a few moments, no-one spoke, each trying to take on board this information. It was complete silence except for the gentle hissing noise from the gas light above them. Tears started trickling down Faith's cheeks.
'I'm sorry, Faith,' Jack said softly, struggling to find the words. 'That's what's been bothering me over these months. You look so much like your mam on this photo and from what I remember of her, you've got her lovely auburn, wavy hair and her greenish-grey eyes; those freckles. John told us that she had a gentle and happy nature, just like you have. When Mary told me that you knew nothing about your dad

apart from his name, I wasn't sure if I should show you this, but it seemed a shame for you not to see it.'

There was another pause. Mary and Tom kept silent. Emma was holding Faith's hand whilst Jack continued with his explanations. 'I started speculating, putting two and two together when I found out the month of your birthday from Emma, as we'd discussed birthdays whilst dancing at Windrush. I was curious to know if it was your dad on the photo. The date was right, plus you mentioned your sister's name once, but I needed more information. When Mary told me about your mam's trip to Seaham and your dad's full name, it was clarification.' Jack pulled out his cigarettes with shaking hands and lit up again.

'Would you two lasses like a shandy?' Tom asked, looking kindly at Faith. 'We've got lemonade.' Faith nodded through her tears, still unable to speak.
'Yes, please, Dad,' answered Emma. 'Can I have a cigarette too.'
'Here, lass, have one of mine,' offered Jack, giving Emma the cigarettes and matches.
'I don't smoke,' ventured Faith, drying her eyes. 'I tried once with my uncles, but it was horrible.' She looked at Jack.
'Thank you for telling me,' she whispered. 'As you know, what you've just told me coincides with information in a letter that my mam wrote just before she died. It will be awhile before it sinks in, but it's lovely to hear someone speak like you have, about my mam. I don't know what else to say. I'm all mixed up.' Her lip was quivering. The tears started rolling. Another silence. No-one knew what to say.
'There's your drink,' said Tom, handing Faith her shandy. 'One for you, Emma, too. It'll be good hay-timing this year when we can have a beer afterwards without walking two miles for it,' he said, cheerily, trying to lighten the situation.

Jack continued, after taking deep breaths.
'I know at the time, John waited and waited, day after day, hoping for a letter from Rose. He used to come in the pub and tell us. He cared about your mam.'
'She wrote,' interrupted Faith. 'My mam, after discovering she was pregnant, but it was about three months later and

the letter was returned *Not at this address.*' Jack looked
downcast.
'John got the offer of a job on another farm over towards the
west coast, plus accommodation, a small cottage. This was
a week before I moved out in late November, the same year.
Unfortunately, we never kept in touch. Shortly after, my
stepdad left to be nearer to his sister. It must have been
after that when your mam wrote.' Faith nodded, trying to
take it all in.

'When did you move to this area? Did you know about your
dad?' Faith asked, trying to deflect the conversation.
'It was early Spring in nineteen forty-one, that I read about
the farm for rent down here after another unpleasant
episode in my life. I decided to move and look for my dad. It
was on her deathbed that mam told me who he was and the
circumstances surrounding her move to Seaham.' Turning to
look at his brother, Jack added, 'That's how I already knew
about you and your family, Tom, before you moved back up
to Bankside, late nineteen forty-two. I found out on the
grapevine.' Returning his attention to Faith, Jack smiled at
her. 'I think I've said enough. I'm glad it's out in the open and
that I've clarified a few things. Would you like this photo as
you're most welcome to it?'
'I would actually. Thank you for telling me. I never thought I'd
see a photo of my dad.' Faith picked up the photo and Jack
handed her the envelope.
'I'm glad that's over with,' Jack stated, taking a deep breath.
'I'll have another pint, Tom, if you don't mind.'

Mary went to settle Miriam as she could hear her
whimpering, just as Tim appeared, grinning from ear to ear,
carrying in a dead rabbit. Martha walked in with a bag of
shopping. Suddenly, everyone was talking as Tim described
his exploits with rabbits and Martha chatted to the two girls
about her trip to Whitby. Tom and Jack finished their pints
and walked out, after Jack said his goodbyes.
'We're going to bed now,' stated Emma, an hour or so later.
Mary said goodnight to Faith, whispering quietly to her.
'What did mam say?' queried Emma, when they were behind
closed doors in the sitting room.
'She said she was pleased that I'd finally got a picture of my

dad, or something like that. She thanked me for being so helpful.' When they were both in bed, Faith shared her feelings. 'I'm trying to take it all in. It's such a bombshell. You know, Emma, I kind of feel I'm not an orphan anymore. I've also got this lovely family who've always made me feel so welcome. I'm a bit overwhelmed, I think.' Emma smiled, not wanting to comment at that moment in case she said the wrong thing. However, this didn't stop the girls talking, well into the night.

After a few more days together, the girls returned to boarding school and intense studying. A couple of weeks into the summer term, the ballroom dancing exam results were announced.
'You have all done extremely well,' stated Mrs Carruthers. 'Come forward as your name is called and you will be presented with your certificate and medal.' The two tutors were on the stage beside her and one gave Emma her certificate and the other, the medal, whilst each congratulated her. Emma and Faith both were awarded a gold medal with the engraved words: *Empire Society. Old Time Dance Test.* On Emma's certificate were the words, *Amateur Test "Olde Tyme"- Ballroom Dancing* and in brackets, after her name, was the word *Commended*.

Emma read the accompanying piece of paper, giving the marks and comments for each individual dance.
'My goodness,' she thought, seeing eighty percent allocated for four of the dances and eighty-two percent for the Royal Empress Tango. 'That's because Mrs Carruthers bent me backwards and forwards, making me do all the actions correctly in The Tango,' she thought, smiling to herself. Then she read the comments, which included: *Try to improve deportment*, written three times and another was: r*elax more*. 'No surprise there,' she acknowledged, remembering how tense she'd been. At the end of the ceremony, following a speech of thanks by Mrs Carruthers, the girls stood and applauded their teacher and the tutors.
'They do the Tango at Windrush dance,' Emma later said to Faith. 'We'll be able to get up and do it together and the Two Step. I'm so glad we went to these classes.'

The results also arrived for the Religious Examination, taken in March. Emma was awarded a pass plus.

'I am surprised, Emma,' stated Mother Colette, handing her the certificate. 'I thought you would have at least obtained a credit. That is a little disappointing.'

'It must have been that question on the cornerstone of the faith,' mused Emma. 'I guess they couldn't give me a higher mark with a blunder like that.' She heard the nun congratulate Faith who was awarded a credit. From then on, it was revision, revision, revision for the GCEs. Mother Colette, being the Latin teacher for their form, was also disappointed at Emma's result in the mock exam.

'Twenty-eight percent, Emma,' she stated. 'That's not good enough. We have a lot of work to do. You can do better than that.'

Night after night, the girls studied and revised. Even in her cubicle in bed, Emma continued, trying to memorise facts. This was possible because the natural light in the evenings extended well past their bedtime at eight-thirty. After putting her revision book on her bedside locker, she opened the drawer and took out a prayer card, the one she'd bought at Walsingham. Not even Faith knew which one she bought. It was a prayer to Saint Jude, well-known as the patron saint of hopeless cases. Emma knew about Saint Jude because when Mary had a bad headache, she used to ask her older children to pray to Saint Jude.

'I'm not a hopeless case,' thought Emma, 'but I need help and if he can help lost causes, then he'll be able to help me.' It was her nightly ritual along with revising.

There was the opportunity, at half-term, for a brief recess from the constant studying. Faith decided to go home as she wanted to see her sister and uncles to show them the photo of her mam and dad.

'I'll have some quiet and rest,' she said to Emma, 'before the final hurdle of exams.'

'Understandably so,' thought Emma, when later at Bankside, she was sitting in her bedroom, trying to work but with interruptions from little siblings who wanted her company. 'Maybe I should have a couple of days off too.'

It was when she was making a cup of tea in the kitchen that Jack Netherfield called in, having come to see Tom.
'I'm glad I've caught you, Emma. I wanted to tell you that Greg has been asking after you. He's taken a shine to you, I think. He wants to know if you will be around in summer.'
'Hello, Uncle Jack. Yes, I'll be here after we break up, but for how long, I don't know, as I will be applying for jobs. Faith is going to join me later in August. We have decided to go into digs together if we can get jobs in the same town. She didn't come this time as she wanted to show that photo you gave her, to her sister and uncles. It was lovely for her, you know, finding it. She keeps it with her all the time. She also went home for some quiet time in order to revise.'
'Well, best of luck to you both with all those exams. I'll see you in the summer.'
'Thanks, Uncle Jack.'

Back at school, Emma studied relentlessly at every opportunity, including break times, at recreation and late into the evenings in bed. She opened her cubicle curtain to make use of the fading light from the window facing her across the narrow corridor. She was tired, but each time she crossed off a subject after taking it, she realised the end was drawing nearer when she would be able to play tennis and read without constantly worrying about studying.

'Emma,' called Mother Colette, coming out of her office as Emma was passing, on her way to the boarders' room, one morning. 'Take these Latin exam papers to the chapel and pray. You need all the help you can get considering how badly you did in your mock exam. Go on, off you go,' she added, putting the sealed manila envelope into Emma's hands. Emma turned and went down the stairs to the vestry. She took her hat from the peg.
'Thank goodness the uniform hat was changed,' she though, placing it on her head. 'These scull-type caps are much better than the larger brown hats with elastic to hold them in place.'

She quietly opened the chapel door and closing it gently after her, crept down the aisle. A couple of elderly nuns were in their pews, mumbling their prayers. Emma went to the front and placing the envelope beside her, knelt and gazed at the crucifix. She didn't say any formal prayers. It was mainly a mental chat about the Latin exam and those taking it. She didn't was to disappoint Mother Colette after her poor performance in the mock exam.

The exams finally came to an end. It was a great relief for the girls especially for the boarders who, although not leaving until term ceased, were allowed more freedom and time out. Pupils in Emma's form, unwinding after their intense few weeks, spent a hilarious day, not in uniform, sitting talking on the convent lawns or fooling about pretending to spray each other with the garden hosepipe. The relief was intense.

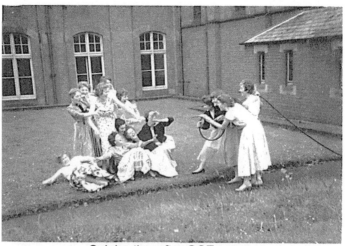

Celebrating after GCE exams

During the period following the end of exams, the upper fifth year pupils were invited to participate in a retreat, but it wasn't compulsory. There were talks and reflective time plus some quiet meditation and prayer times. On the Saturday evening, Father White, one of the priests helping, invited the handful of boarders, making the retreat, to an informal discussion period. This was something different on a Saturday night and the girls decided to give it a go. They met up in the domestic science room.

'Is this young lady going to follow in your footsteps, Mother Colette?' the priest asked, as Emma was approaching them at the doorway of the room. The headmistress smiled.
'No, I don't think so. I think the other side is uppermost in Emma. Enjoy your evening, Father,' she added, as she left.
The priest followed Emma into the room. She was deliberating over Mother Colette's comment.
'I suppose she means marriage and children,' Emma mused. 'I remember once thinking about being a nun but only if I could go to Africa and look after those little black babies that we collected pennies for, when I was at primary school. Maybe I will get married and have lots of children.' She thought she'd enjoy that.

The priest explained that everything said was to be treated confidentially and not to go beyond the room. One of the girls opened the windows as it was such a warm evening. They sat around in a small circle and Father White asked them about their plans and their hobbies. He was a good facilitator, very gentle and non-judgemental. Gradually, everyone relaxed and began chatting, revealing problems and concerns. The discussion turned to relationships and feeling at ease, the girls were quite forthcoming about boyfriends. They were growing up. The priest admitted to smoking and pulled out a packet of cigarettes.
'Anyone here smoke?' he questioned. 'I bet some of you do. No-one is going to tell.' The girls looked at each other.
'I do sometimes,' Emma offered, 'when I go to dances at home with my sister. When we helped at hay time last summer, we smoked with our dad, sitting under the hedgerow, taking a break. He smokes woodbines. My mam does as well.' There was a slight pause before another girl put up her hand and admitted that she, too, smoked occasionally.
'Thank you for your honesty,' commented the priest. 'It takes courage to own up to doing something that may not be approved of, by others.'

He opened the packet and taking one out, broke it in two and gave the two smokers a half each.
'Thank you,' they replied, as he offered them a light. Emma was grinning.

'Fancy having a smoke on retreat and in a convent at that. Who would have imagined it?' she thought.

'Just a reminder,' Father White continued. 'We keep this to ourselves.' The girls nodded. They continued chatting for another three quarters of an hour before he closed the meeting with a prayer. His final request was to ask the girls to each complete a form with feedback which, he explained, may help when giving his next retreat.

'It feels like we're really growing up, filling in that questionnaire,' commented Faith, as the girls made their way to the dormitory.

The end of term was fast approaching, but a final challenge arose for Emma when Audrey decided to have a midnight feast in the dormitory.

'We have worked hard. We've finished our exams. It's not as if we can be expelled,' she reasoned, to the other five boarders in her year group. Most of us are leaving for good at the end of this term. What can they do to us? Nothing! Let's celebrate.' She went around quietly whispering the plans. Emma was reluctant to join in. She felt there were limits on how many rules should be broken. Food in the dormitory was forbidden as was talking without permission. As for climbing over cubicle partitions in the middle of the night, that was a big one and Emma didn't want to damage unduly her good reputation at this late stage of her boarding school years.

'You are coming, aren't you?' Faith asked her, later in the evening. 'You know. What Audrey has planned, for Tuesday night.' She nodded. She didn't feel able to refuse.

Luckily, Audrey's cubicle was on the inner aisle, back to back with Emma's on the garden side. She only had to climb over. With her heart in her mouth, in the pitch darkness and being as quiet as possible, she scaled the cubicle top by standing on the bedside cabinet, heaving herself over and landing onto Audrey's bed. Already three other girls were there. They'd sneaked out and crept around to Audrey's, passing Mother Teresa's cubicle on the way. They were amazed at their audacity. They whispered and giggled quietly, whilst drinking juice supplied by Audrey and munching on biscuits and sweets.

'We can always tell our children that we had a midnight feast at boarding school,' whispered Rita, who'd arrived a short while later. Emma said little. She was petrified at being found out.

Eventually, leaving Audrey's cubicle, one at a time, they crept stealthily back to their beds. This time, Emma went up the aisle and back to garden side, thankful that no-one had been caught. The girls gave knowing smiles to one another, over breakfast next morning, not daring to believe that they'd got away with it. They were expecting to be called out at any moment, but it seemed that this time, luck was on their side. Emma wondered if Mother Teresa had heard them and turned a blind eye, or ear in this case. It was, she decided, quite a good way to finish five years of boarding school.

School finally ended. Emma packed her case for the last time. She didn't know how to get her bedding home, but Mary told her to leave it for the nuns as she was sure they'd find a use for it. The final sing song wasn't too upsetting as they had all their futures to look forward to. She was excited because Faith was going to join her after returning home to await the GCE results being forwarded to them in August. They were planning to apply for jobs in the civil service together. Mother Colette asked for self-addressed postcards from each boarder who had taken exams, so that she could write down their results and post them. Certificates would be received a later date.
'And while we wait for those,' Emma said to Faith, 'I will have fun at home and go to dances weekly.' They were interrupted by the bell ringing. 'Bedtime at half eight for the last time! Yippee,' she thought. She couldn't wait.

'I'm here, Mam,' called Emma, walking into the farmhouse kitchen.
'She's getting the washing in,' stated Amy, getting up and giving her big sister a hug. Emma bent down to pick up Miriam.
'You are so lovely and cute.'
'Aren't you getting tall,' she said to Amy.
'If I pass my scholarship next year, I'm going to the convent school, like you,' Amy replied. 'Mark and Jacob are outside

somewhere, larking about. I think dad went to Uncle Jack's to help him with some job or other. You are in the sitting room, like you always are. Martha went to Whitby, but she should be back soon.'

'Just like old times,' thought Emma, carrying her case into the sitting room. 'I'll have two drawers,' she thought, looking at the small four drawer chest near the bed. She unpacked and changed and went through to the kitchen.

'Hello,' called her mother, coming from the back kitchen. 'I'm putting the kettle on, if you want a cup of tea.' At that moment, the door opened and Tom walked in. He gave Emma a hug.

'I'll have a drink as well, Mary, if there's enough water in the kettle.'

'Well, lass, what does it feel like to have left?' Tom asked, whilst sitting for ten minutes with his mug of tea.

'It's great, Dad. Did mam tell you that Faith and I are applying for jobs once our results are through. I hope they will be good enough. We thought we might find work in the same town so that we can share digs.'

'Aye, she said you'd written about it. You two will do fine. Clever lasses like you. We'll get a bit of work out of you before you go, though,' he added, jokingly, 'won't we, Mary?' Her mother smiled.

'You can start by sorting out your clothes, if you like,' she said to Emma. 'The little ones need a bath tonight. You'll enjoy that. It's baking day tomorrow as we're about out of cakes. I love it when you come home and do the weekly bake.'

'I'll need help with the hay and there's plenty of weeding to do,' Tom added. Then her parents smiled.

'Don't worry. There will be plenty of time for dancing. You and Martha can have some fun together,' reassured Mary, seeing the serious look on Emma's face. 'It won't be work all the time.'

It was well into August before the postman delivered Emma's postcard on which, clearly written, were her exam results.

'Well?' asked Mary, waiting for her daughter to tell her. It was mid-afternoon and Tom was at Whitby, shopping.

Emma was beaming.
'I have passed them all. Latin, French, Spanish, English Literature, English language, Maths, Geography and Biology. I can't believe it.' She felt light-headed and mentally said a prayer of thanks especially to Saint Jude as she'd been given fifty-five percent for her Latin. Her best mark was for English Language, followed by English Literature, but passing them all was just unbelievable; Emma's head was spinning. 'I think I might just cry,' she said, suddenly feeling very emotional and tearful. Mary gave her a hug.
'I'm happy for you, Emma. Well done. All that hard work has paid off. Your dad will be pleased. Now you'll be able to put the results on an application form when you apply for jobs. Mind you, when your dad gets to know, he might talk you into going back to do 'A' levels, with doing so well.
'Thanks, Mam. It's difficult to take in,' replied Emma. 'I wonder if Faith passed all hers. I hope so.'

Very early next morning, waking up at dawn with the cock crowing and unable to go back to sleep, unlike Martha lying sleeping beside her, Emma was thinking.
'Five years ago, I was that timid, nervous, frightened little girl trying to adapt to a strange existence totally unlike anything I'd been used to. Look at me now.' She realised that she'd received a good academic education but more than that, she'd developed and matured into a confident young adult.
'Having some understanding teachers and friends, especially Faith, helped me,' Emma acknowledged, 'as well as the security of a loving family. Although it was difficult in those early years, I came through and if it is a question in life, of sink or swim, then I am going to swim no matter what challenges lay ahead.' Emma smiled.

Ingram Content Group UK Ltd.
Milton Keynes UK
UKHW010122190523
421862UK00015B/23